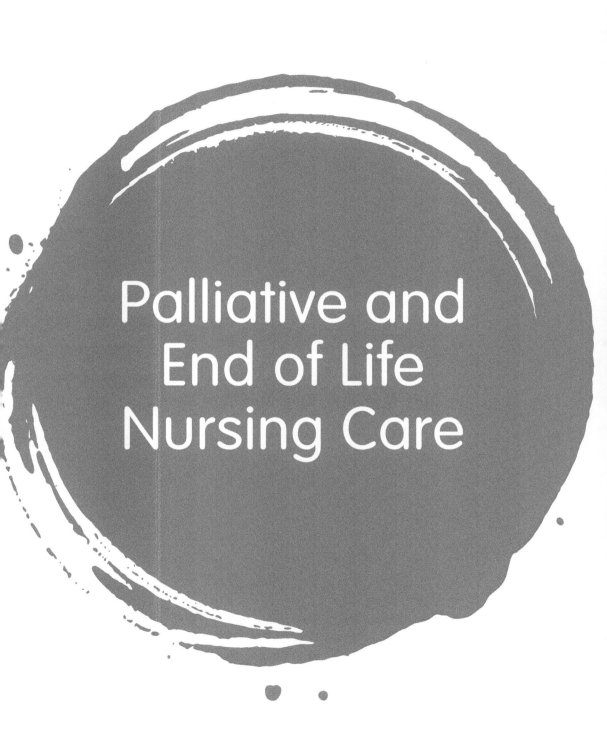

Palliative and End of Life Nursing Care

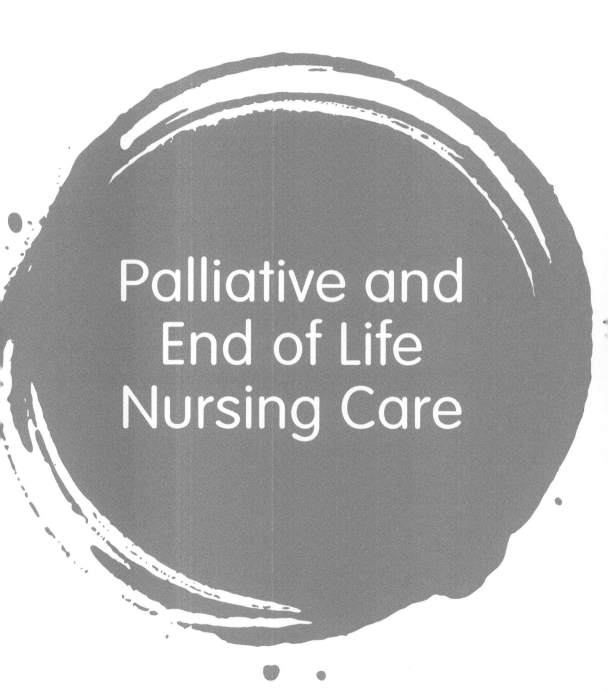

Palliative and End of Life Nursing Care

Beth Hardy
Kate Flemming

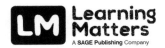

Learning Matters
A SAGE Publishing Company
1 Oliver's Yard
55 City Road
London EC1Y 1SP

SAGE Publications Inc.
2455 Teller Road
Thousand Oaks, California 91320

SAGE Publications India Pvt Ltd
B 1/I 1 Mohan Cooperative Industrial Area
Mathura Road
New Delhi 110 044

SAGE Publications Asia-Pacific Pte Ltd
3 Church Street
#10-04 Samsung Hub
Singapore 049483

Editor: Martha Cunneen
Development editor: Sarah Turpie
Senior project editor: Chris Marke
Marketing manager: Ruslana Khatagova
Cover design: Sheila Tong
Typeset by: C&M Digitals (P) Ltd, Chennai, India

Library of Congress Control Number: 2023930608

British Library Cataloguing in Publication Data

A catalogue record for this book is available from the
British Library

ISBN 978-1-5297-7150-3
ISBN 978-1-5297-7151-0 (pbk)

Contents

Acknowledgements   viii
About the authors   ix

Introduction   1

1   The changing face of palliative and end of life care   6

2   Person-centred and cultural considerations for care   23

3   Expected deaths   40

4   Living with advanced life-limiting illness   61

5   Complexity in palliative and end of life care   81

6   Planning for the end of life   101

7   Families and carers   119

8   Research and evidence-based practice in palliative and end of life care   136

Glossary   155
References   157
Index   168

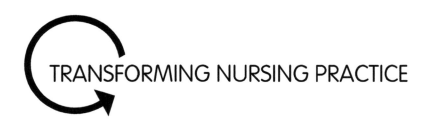

TRANSFORMING NURSING PRACTICE

Transforming Nursing Practice is a series tailor made for pre-registration student nurses. Each book in the series is:

✓ Affordable

✓ Full of active learning features

✓ Mapped to the NMC Standards of proficiency for registered nurses

✓ Focused on applying theory to practice

Each book addresses a core topic and they have been carefully developed to be simple to use, quick to read and written in clear language.

An invaluable series of books that explicitly relates to the NMC standards. Each book covers a different topic that students need to explore in order to develop into a qualified nurse... I would recommend this series to all Pre-Registered nursing students whatever their field or year of study.

LINDA ROBSON,
Senior Lecturer at Edge Hill University

Many titles in the series are on our recommended reading list and for good reason - the content is up to date and easy to read. These are the books that actually get used beyond training and into your nursing career.

EMMA LYDON,
Adult Student Nursing

ABOUT THE SERIES EDITORS

DR MOOI STANDING is an Independent Nursing Consultant (UK and International) and is responsible for the core knowledge, adult nursing and personal and professional learning skills titles. She is an experienced NMC Quality Assurance Reviewer of educational programmes and a Professional Regulator Panellist on the NMC Practice Committee. Mooi is also Board member of Special Olympics Malaysia, enabling people with intellectual disabilities to participate in sports and athletics nationally and internationally.

DR SANDRA WALKER is a Clinical Academic in Mental Health working between Southern Health Trust and the University of Southampton and responsible for the mental health nursing titles. She is a Qualified Mental Health Nurse with a wide range of clinical experience spanning more than 25 years.

BESTSELLING TEXTBOOKS

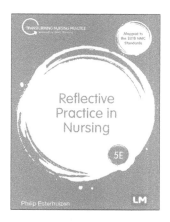

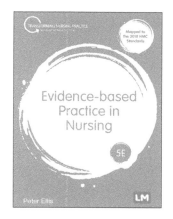

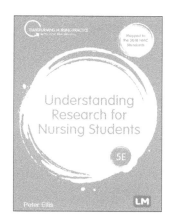

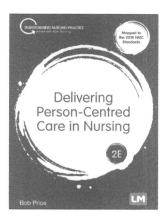

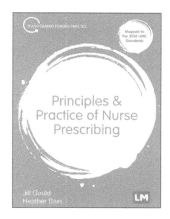

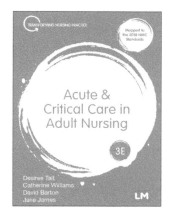

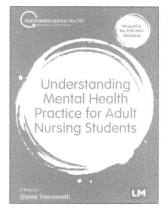

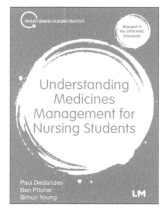

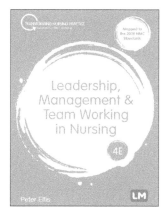

You can find a full list of textbooks in the *Transforming Nursing Practice* series at

https://uk.sagepub.com/TNP-series

Acknowledgements

We were guided in writing this textbook by an advisory group of undergraduate student nurses. Their commitment to care for people facing the end of life and their enthusiasm for sharing ideas and collaborating with each other was inspiring and helped shape the contents of this text. Betty Owino, Dee Duncan-Cottingham, Kate Grainger, Kheira Haffiane, Nisha Reynolds, Lizzie Cunningham and Natasha Tomblin: Thank you.

We are also grateful to Clair Fisher for the discussions about complexity in healthcare and so candidly sharing her experiences of facing the end of life; Sean Collins, Managing Director at The Like Minded (www.thelikeminded.co.uk/) for supplying the images for the 'how to' guide of 'What matters' conversation in Chapter 7; Kate Rudd and Amanda Whateley for peer review and feedback; and the team at SAGE Learning Matters for their support throughout this process.

Dr Beth Hardy and Professor Kate Flemming

About the Authors

Beth Hardy is a Senior Lecturer in Nursing at the University of York and a Queen's Nurse. Before entering academia, Beth worked as a district nurse. Her experiences of delivering end of life care in the community have fuelled her interest in dying and death and in educational approaches that prepare student nurses to provide palliative and end of life care.

Kate Flemming is an experienced academic and nurse, internationally known for her leading research and service innovation in palliative care nursing. Kate leads by example through her pioneering clinical leadership and research in palliative care within the hospice and community settings. Kate works in the Department of Health Sciences at the University of York where she is a Professor of Hospice Practice and Evidence Synthesis.

Introduction

Who is this book for?

This book is an introduction to palliative and end of life nursing care for adults. It is aimed specifically at students studying to become a nurse but may also be of interest to registered nurses looking to refresh their knowledge and students studying on other health professions programmes such as nursing associate, medicine and the allied professions. The book aims to support you to develop competence and confidence in palliative and end of life care and to understand key concepts and principles that underpin this. It is written by experts in the field, with guidance from current student nurses, all of whom have a passion for palliative and end of life care and have drawn on their own learning experiences to support the development of the text.

Why palliative and end of life nursing care?

At some point in their career, all nurses, regardless of their field of practice, will be involved with the care of people living with life-limiting and advanced illness, those facing the end of their lives, and the families and carers that are connected to them. Care will occur in multiple settings, which include those where people are accessing support for needs relating to their palliative and/or end of life care, but also those where they seek support for other needs that coexist with their life-limiting illnesses. These locations will include people's homes, hospitals, residential and nursing homes, hospices, general practice, mental health facilities, out-patient clinics and specialist services for people with learning disabilities. Awareness and understanding of the challenges faced by people who have life-limiting illness and who are facing the end of their life is needed by all nurses. The way that nursing care is provided towards the end of life will make a significant difference to people's experiences during this time and to their quality of life.

Working with people who have advanced life-limiting illnesses, or who are dying, can be some of the most challenging elements of nursing practice. Nurses need to reflect on their own experiences, thoughts and feelings about death and explore how these may impact on their interactions with people and the nursing care that they provide. They also need to develop strategies to maintain their own wellbeing to ensure they can maintain standards of care while protecting their own health. Equally, working with people in these circumstances can be some of the most rewarding elements of nursing practice, with opportunity to influence and improve the lives of patients, families and carers.

Underpinning good care requires nurses to draw on their broad nursing knowledge and skills and develop specific knowledge of the support needs of people with advanced life-limiting illness, the palliative approach to care and of care in the last days of life. This book focuses on the specific knowledge required.

Book structure

The book is structured to guide your learning, so if you are new to learning about palliative and end of life care we suggest reading it in the order it is written. If you already have some underpinning knowledge and have focused learning goals you may want to go specifically to the chapter that addresses these – for example, if you are particularly wanting to develop your knowledge of supporting families and carers then this is covered in Chapter 7.

We have placed people at the heart of this textbook: patients, families and healthcare staff are at the core of palliative and end of life care. The first section of the book (Chapters 1 and 2) explores approaches to care. We discuss important theoretical considerations which will develop your understanding of palliative and person-centred care and your knowledge of why this matters when you are working with people living with life-limiting illness. The second section of the book (Chapters 3–7) explores what happens to people as they approach the end of their lives, and ways that you can support patients and their families through this period. Finally, we explore how the evidence base for palliative and end of life care is developed, and your role in using the evidence to underpin your practice. We discuss the chapters in more detail below.

Chapter 1, The changing face of palliative and end of life care: The book starts by exploring the key concepts of palliative and end of life care, and what these terms mean. We consider how end of life care has changed over the years and how care is currently provided.

Chapter 2, Person-centred and cultural considerations for care: In this chapter, we explore person-centred care and consider the relationship between this concept and relationship-centred care. We discuss how someone's personhood and their sense of identity may be affected by their illness, and explore cultural competence and the significance of this for nursing practice. We will also consider inequity in access to palliative care.

Chapter 3, Expected deaths: This chapter introduces you to commonly seen signs that someone is likely to be dying and explores what dying might be like from patient, family and nurse perspectives. We discuss the concept of a 'good death' and invite you to reflect on your own feelings and thoughts about death and dying. It includes 'top tips' for working with people during the last days of their lives, which were suggested by our student advisory group.

Chapter 4, Living with advanced life-limiting illness: Palliative care is about helping people to live as well as they can in their circumstances. This chapter will consider what 'health' means when someone is living with incurable illness, explores factors that contribute to living well and the importance of identifying people's personal goals for care. We will also consider the role of symptom management in a palliative approach to care.

Chapter 5, Complexity in palliative and end of life care: This chapter will explore what is meant by 'complexity', and factors that contribute to people having complex support needs. We will examine the role of specialist palliative care and you will be encouraged to identify your personal strategies for self-care and reflect on how you may develop and maintain these.

Chapter 6, Planning for the end of life: In this chapter we consider why and how people might plan for their end of life and introduce you to some processes that relate to this. This includes advance care planning, advance decisions to refuse treatment (ADRT), do not attempt cardiopulmonary resuscitation (DNACPR) orders and lasting power of attorney (LPA).

Chapter 7, Families and carers: The palliative approach to care explicitly considers the support needs of families and carers, alongside those of the patient. We will discuss the role that families and carers take in supporting people living with life-limiting conditions and at the end of life and consider the impact of caring on carers and the role of services to support them.

Chapter 8, Research and evidence-based practice in palliative and end of life care: Finally, this chapter discusses the role of research and of evidence-based practice in palliative care. This includes looking at some of the challenges of undertaking research in this area and considering your role in developing the evidence base and in using evidence for safe and effective practice.

Requirements for the NMC *Standards of Proficiency for Registered Nurses*

The Nursing and Midwifery Council (NMC) has established standards of proficiency to be met by applicants to different parts of the register, and these are the standards it considers necessary for safe and effective practice. This book is structured so that it will help you to understand and meet the proficiencies required for entry to the NMC register. The relevant proficiencies are presented at the start of each chapter so that you can clearly see which ones the chapter addresses. The proficiencies have been designed to be generic so apply to all fields of nursing and all care settings. This is because all nurses must be able to meet the needs of any person they encounter in their practice regardless of their stage of life or health challenges, whether these are mental, physical, cognitive or behavioural.

This book includes the latest standards for 2018 onwards, taken from the *Future Nurse: Standards of Proficiency for Registered Nurses* (NMC, 2018).

Learning features

Learning from reading text is not always easy. Therefore, to provide variety and to assist with the development of independent learning skills and the application of theory to practice, this book contains activities, case studies, scenarios, further reading, useful websites and other materials to enable you to participate in your own learning. You will need to develop your own study skills and 'learn how to learn' to get the best from the material. The book cannot provide all the answers – but instead provides a framework for your learning.

The activities in the book will in particular help you to make sense of, and learn about, the material being presented. Some activities ask you to reflect on aspects of practice, or your experience of it, or the people or situations you encounter. Reflection is an essential skill in nursing, and it helps you to understand the world around you and often to identify how things might be improved. Communication is fundamental in palliative care and activities will help you to think about your communication skills and to develop these. Other activities will help you develop key graduate skills such as your ability to think critically about a topic in order to challenge received wisdom, or your ability to research a topic and find appropriate information and evidence, and to be able to make decisions using that evidence in situations that are often difficult and time-pressured.

All the activities require you to take a break from reading the text, think through the issues presented and carry out some independent study, possibly using the internet. Where appropriate there are sample answers presented at the end of each chapter and these will help you to understand more fully your own reflections and independent study. Remember, academic study will always require independent work and these activities will help to deepen your knowledge and understanding of the issues under scrutiny and give you practice at working on your own.

You might want to think about completing these activities as part of your personal development plan (PDP) or portfolio. After completing the activity, write it up in your PDP or portfolio in a section devoted to that particular skill, then look back over time to see how far you are developing. You can also do more of the activities for a key skill that you have identified a weakness in, which will help build your skill and confidence in this area.

This book also contains a glossary on page 155 to assist you with unfamiliar terms. Glossary terms are in bold in the first instance that they appear.

We hope you enjoy reading this book as much as we enjoyed writing it. As nurses and academics we are both passionate about providing high-quality palliative and end of life care. We hope through our writing that we are able to pass on some of our passion and enthusiasm to you, to support you in caring for patients, and their families, at the end of their lives.

Chapter 1 The changing face of palliative and end of life care

Chapter aims

After reading this chapter, you will:

- be able to define the key concepts of dying, palliative care and end of life care
- have knowledge about the history and development of palliative care
- understand the role of the nurse in caring for people with life-limiting conditions and for people who are dying, and their families
- understand that there are many different locations where end of life care can be delivered
- appreciate that end of life care is relevant to all nursing roles.

Case study: Isaac

Isaac was coming towards the end of his second-year placement on an acute medical ward. During his placement he had really enjoyed the variety of experiences he had gained working on a general ward. Many of the people he had cared for had been admitted onto the ward acutely unwell but had recovered sufficiently during their stay to be discharged home and would be able to resume their previous lives. Isaac was aware though, that a small number of people on the ward needed palliative care and were nearing the end of their lives. Due to his shift patterns, Isaac hadn't had much opportunity to be involved in the care of these patients, but he did know that some had been discharged from the ward to a hospice, some had gone home with rapidly arranged additional support and other people had died while on the ward. Isaac was interested to know more about palliative care and whether this was different to end of life care, and how many people actually died in hospitals.

Introduction

Dying is a normal part of human life and as a student nurse, you will be involved with the care of people who are living with a diagnosis of a **life-limiting illness** and those who are at the **end of life**. Nurses in some roles will specifically focus on this type of care, while others will only occasionally work with patients and families facing the end of life. **Palliative care** occurs in many care settings and knowing about palliative care will enable you to appropriately support patients and their families as they access, and transition between, care services – for example, between hospital and home which was the situation for some patients on the acute medical ward where Isaac was on placement. These transitions between care settings occur in other contexts as well – for example, people who use mental health or learning disability services also have other health support needs and will, at some point, also die. Regardless of your field of practice, knowledge of palliative care is important.

This chapter will introduce you to core concepts that we discuss throughout this book: palliative and end of life care. We will consider the differing roles generalist and specialist services have in caring for people life-limiting illnesses. We explore the history and development of palliative and end of life care to give you some understanding of how services have evolved, as well as introducing you to Dame Cicely Saunders, a pivotal figure in the development of palliative care and inspiring woman who fought to improve the lives of people who were dying. We then move on to consider the various ways in which nurses provide care to people who are nearing the end of their lives and encourage you to reflect on your own observations of nursing practice. Finally, we will consider the data available which describes where people die, the kind of locations where palliative and end of life care is delivered and what may change in the future.

What is palliative care?

The care of people who are nearing the end of their lives or who are dying has always been central to a nurse's role. The origins of end of life nursing care began through the work of Mary Seacole and Florence Nightingale during the mid-1800s in the Crimean War, with the nursing processes they introduced having an impact on the quality of life and death for those injured. However, while we can trace back the early principles of end of life nursing care to over 200 years ago, what we know of as 'modern' palliative care today is something that has developed over the last few decades.

Palliative care is an **holistic** approach to the care of people with life-limiting illness, their families and/or those who are close to them. Its origins can be understood from the word 'palliate' which is defined as *To alleviate (a disease or its symptoms) without effecting a cure; to relieve or ease (physical or emotional suffering) temporarily or superficially* (Oxford English Dictionary, 2022), or 'to cloak', as in to cover or mask symptoms. It is a clinical speciality that is known internationally and has been defined by the World Health Organization.

Concept summary: World Health Organization definition of palliative care

Palliative care is an approach that improves the quality of life of patients (adults and children) and their families who are facing problems associated with life-threatening illness. It prevents and relieves suffering through the early identification, correct assessment and treatment of pain and other problems, whether physical, psychosocial, or spiritual.

Addressing suffering involves taking care of issues beyond physical symptoms. Palliative care uses a team approach to support patients and their caregivers. This includes addressing practical needs and providing bereavement counselling. It offers a support system to help patients live as actively as possible until death. Palliative care is explicitly recognized under the human right to health. It should be provided through person-centered and integrated health services that pay special attention to the specific needs and preferences of individuals.

Palliative care is required for a wide range of diseases. Most adults in need of palliative care have chronic diseases such as cardiovascular diseases, cancer, chronic respiratory diseases, AIDS and diabetes. Many other conditions may require palliative care, including kidney failure, chronic liver disease, multiple sclerosis, Parkinson's disease, rheumatoid arthritis, neurological disease, dementia, congenital anomalies and drug-resistant tuberculosis.

World Health Organization (2022)

Palliative care is an approach to care that is applicable to all fields of nursing practice including adult, learning disability, child and mental health. As an undergraduate nurse, you are likely to care for people who require palliative care across many different placement settings. Palliative care can occur in people's own homes, nursing and residential homes, hospitals and in hospices; a palliative approach to care can be considered in any setting where a person is living with a life-limiting illness.

A palliative approach to care is one that seeks to maximise an individual's quality of life as they live with and die from a life-limiting illness. It adopts a comfort-focused approach to care, seeking to minimise the impact of physical, psychological and/or spiritual symptoms that an individual may be experiencing. Sometimes, it will be offered alongside **curative care**. Care of those people who are significant to the person who is unwell is a further key component of palliative care; this may be either family members, friends or both. For simplicity, in this book, we use the expression 'family' to capture these significant relationships despite their different named relationships. Those closest to the individual may additionally take on the role of informal carer during the final stages of the illness, and the needs of these people who are providing care are vital. We explore the experiences of families and informal carers and how best to provide support in more detail in Chapter 7.

One of the most challenging aspects of palliative care can be determining when in the progress of their illness someone may benefit from palliative care. Looking at the list of diseases contained within the WHO (2022) definition of palliative care above, it might seem simple to work out who might benefit from palliative care, if it was decided by diagnosis alone. However, different illnesses can take different courses, or trajectories, and people respond in different ways to living with illness, which can make predicting when someone may benefit from receiving palliative care more difficult. Different disease trajectories are discussed in more detail in Chapter 4.

It is helpful to look at what is meant by the terms 'palliative care' and 'end of life' in relation to time frames of illness; both may be terms you have heard used in practice. End of life is often used to refer to the last few hours, days or weeks of life (where people are often also referred to as 'dying'). This can be hard to predict with certainty and we consider this further in Chapter 3 where we explore 'expected deaths'.

Palliative care is used to refer to the approach to care we described above, which may be delivered for months or years leading up to the person's death, depending on the circumstances of the patient. There is, however, some inconsistency in terminology, which can cause confusion. A number of key NHS policy documents refer to end of life care as the last twelve months of life (Department of Health, 2008; NHS Long Term Plan, 2019). These documents suggest that end of life care planning should, where feasible, commence for people who are expected to die within the next twelve months, but acknowledge that this will be dependent on the individual, their personal circumstances and those of their illness. Because of this inconsistency, when you come across these terms while you are on placement it is important to establish how they are being used.

Whatever terminology is used, the principles of palliative care are embedded in end of life care. As highlighted, the focus of this care is to enable someone with an advanced life-limiting illness to live as well as possible until they die. This includes supporting the needs of the patient and their family/friends, and having a plan to support their care in an holistic way (Leadership Alliance for the Care of Dying People (LACDP), 2014).

In this book, we use the term 'end of life' to refer to the final period of life which is anticipated to be weeks, days or hours, and palliative care to refer to an approach to care which is applicable to anyone living with a life-limiting illness. The following activity (1.1) invites you to consider your current knowledge of palliative care.

Activity 1.1 Critical thinking

Think about the following questions:

1. What do you currently know about palliative care?
2. Where have you heard this term?
3. Is palliative care only for people who are expected to die soon?

No answer is given to the first two questions of this activity as it is based on your own knowledge and experiences. An answer to the third question is given at the end of the chapter.

Generalist and specialist palliative care

In Activity 1.1 you reflected on your current understanding of palliative care and you may have identified that you have heard the phrase 'palliative care' in hospital and community settings. While we have discussed that a palliative approach to care is relevant to most healthcare settings, it is worth noting that there are different ways that palliative care is organised. Palliative care can be delivered as part of generalist services (also sometimes called universal care services) – that is, it is available and embedded within other services such as an acute hospital and also as a specialist service in its own right. We will look at each of these in turn.

Generalist palliative care

The majority of palliative care that people receive is delivered as part of generalist palliative care. Generalist palliative care is provided by health professionals whose role is providing care to people with a range of problems and support needs across the life span. Palliative care is just one component of their work. These health professionals will work in a variety of settings including general practice, people's own homes, nursing homes and acute and community hospitals, and include general practitioners (GPs), district and community nurses, hospital-based nurses and healthcare assistants. They may have received some education and training in palliative and end of life care and integrate this learning into their broader role. This enables such individuals to deliver palliative care in a way that is integrated into their usual practice. Those working in generalist palliative care will often receive support from specialist palliative care practitioners.

Specialist palliative care

Specialist palliative care is required by a smaller number of people who have more complex palliative care needs, such as those with symptoms which may be challenging to manage or have social, emotional or psychological needs that are best supported by a specialist. It is provided by specialist palliative care teams, which are multidisciplinary and whose staff have received specialist training. The whole focus of the service, and the people who work within it, is palliative care. These teams can be based in a variety of settings. Most acute hospitals have a specialist palliative care team who support the provision of palliative care across the hospital wards and help to support discharge plans to ensure that if people are able to go home their care is coordinated. Some specialists are community-based, providing specialist palliative care in people's homes and support to those working in general practice and community nursing teams. Most hospices are classed as specialist palliative care units which can provide in-patient, day care and community-based services, led by nursing, allied health professional and medical staff with specialist palliative care training. Specialist palliative care advice provided by these individuals should be readily accessible to health professionals working in settings providing generalist palliative care. Specialist palliative care is a relatively new discipline, becoming a medical speciality in the UK in 1987 – the first country in the world to have this (Clark, 2010). We will explore the role of specialist palliative care further in Chapter 5, where we will consider complexity in palliative and end life care.

Activity 1.2 invites you to reflect back on a clinical placement and the approaches to care you may have experienced for people who are nearing the end of their life.

Activity 1.2 Reflection

Reflect on a time in placement when you have cared for someone who was nearing the end of their life. Was a palliative approach to their care taken? Was this a generalist or specialist approach (or both)? If a palliative approach was not taken, might this care have been beneficial? Why?

As this question is based on your own reflections, there is no answer provided.

Hospice care

In Activity 1.2, you considered your experiences of care for someone nearing the end of life in practice. **Hospice** care is an example of a specialist approach to care. Most towns and cities across the UK have a hospice which provides palliative and end of life care services. There are over 220 hospices across the UK which provide specialist support for either adults or children and young people who have a life-limiting illness. Care in hospices is provided free, and while some funding comes from the NHS (and levels of this vary from hospice to hospice) the majority of funding for hospices comes from charitable donations.

Hospices provide a wide variety of services to support people with life-limiting conditions and those close to them. Most hospices (but not all) have an in-patient unit that will provide care for people in the very last days of life, those who require support with physical or psychological symptoms prior to being discharged home, or who may require respite care for a short period. Many hospices also provide a 'hospice at home' service. This is specialist palliative care provided by hospice practitioners in the person's own home; often these staff work alongside community nurses and GPs. Hospices may also provide a day care provision, where people can come for assessment, symptom management support, access to psychological and complementary therapies on an out-patient basis, often with the support of hospice-provided transport to ease the burden of getting to the hospice. Many hospices also deliver bereavement support services for both the family and friends of people who have died in their care, and the wider community.

Increasingly, hospices are developing outreach services to ensure everyone who requires high-quality palliative care has **equitable** access to it. There are a wide range of individuals and groups who it is known struggle to obtain equitable access to high-quality palliative and end of life care. Hospices are seeking to understand these barriers to ensure services reach and are accessible to those who need them most. These include people from ethnic minority backgrounds, those living in rural communities, those living with frailty and old age, traveller communities, people from the LGBTQ+ community, people with mental health concerns, those who are homeless or vulnerably housed and those who are in prison (Hospice UK, 2021). We will explore some of these issues in more depth in Chapter 2.

Early history of hospices

The term 'hospice' dates back to the Middle Ages in Europe, when it denoted places of charitable refuge offering rest and refreshment to pilgrims and travellers. The development of hospices in the form where they cared for people who were sick and dying began within religious establishments across Europe. The first hospice was developed in the 1600s by a French priest, who founded a nursing order with the purpose of caring for the sick and dying called the Sisters of Charity. Over 200 years later, Our Lady's Hospice was founded in Dublin in 1879. The pace of development then quickened and, in 1891, the first hospice opened in London, known then as the Hostel of God, which still exists today in its modern form as Trinity Hospice in Clapham. Less than ten years later St Joseph's Hospice was founded in the East End of London. It was with the development of St Joseph's that the modern hospice movement began with the work of Dr Cicely Saunders.

Dr Cicely Saunders

Dr Cicely Saunders (who later became Dame Cicely Saunders) is credited with establishing hospice care as we know it today, commonly called the 'modern hospice movement'; it was Cicely Saunders who developed the first 'modern' hospice with St Christopher's Hospice in Sydenham, South London. Cicely Saunders began her career in healthcare as a nurse, but having injured her back she retrained as a hospital almoner (now known as a social worker). During her work in both roles, she encountered people who were dying with poor management of their symptoms, experiencing high levels of distress and who were commonly isolated from other patients, staff and their family. These experiences provided the motivation for Cicely Saunders to seek to improve the care of people who were dying.

She was advised, however, that she would never be able to truly change practice in her role as a hospital almoner, and that she should train as a medical doctor as it is *the doctors who desert the dying* (Oliver, 2015). Undeterred, Cicely Saunders embarked on her medical training and, on qualifying in 1957, studied pain management of people who were dying at St Mary's Hospital, Paddington, while assisting at St Joseph's Hospice. She used her medical expertise and research findings to help the nuns improve their standard of care. Around this time she also published six articles on care of the dying in *Nursing Times*.

Cicely Saunders began to plan and fundraise to build the modern hospice she had dreamed of: a hospice that had a commitment to clinical care, teaching and research. In 1967, Dr Saunders opened the world-renowned St Christopher's Hospice in Sydenham and she became medical director. It was in this role that Cicely Saunders pioneered the use of oral opioid medication to control pain and employed a research assistant, Dr Robert Twycross, to oversee randomised controlled trials testing their effectiveness. As such, Cicely Saunders was pivotal in ensuring that research was a key component underpinning the development of palliative care as a clinical speciality; this continues today.

At St Christopher's, Cicely Saunders also established physician-training programmes to ensure that others could learn about palliative medicine and formulated the basic principles of hospice care, including vigilant attention to patient care. Alongside this she developed the concept of total pain to describe the all-encompassing physical, emotional, spiritual and social distress experienced by many dying patients.

St Christopher's Hospice continues to be one of the most influential hospices in the world, with a robust programme of teaching and research while providing specialist palliative care to those who need it most. Cicely Saunders was made a Dame in 1980 and died in the hospice she founded in 2005.

The following activity invites you to explore hospice services in your local area.

Activity 1.3   Exploring practice

Many towns and cities have a hospice that offers palliative and end of life care services. As a student nurse it is helpful for you to know what services are available locally for the people you care for who are receiving palliative care and/or who are the end of life. Hospice UK (the national charity for hospices) provides a hospice care finder:

https://www.hospiceuk.org/hospice-care-finder/

Use the hospice care finder to locate what hospice and palliative care services are available in your local area.

There are no answers to this activity as it is based on your own investigation.

The role of the nurse in caring for people who are nearing the end of life

So far, we have looked in some detail at the kind of care services that are available for people who are nearing the end of their life and considered how services have developed. We will now consider the role of nurses in caring for people nearing the end of their lives. The following activity invites you to reflect on your role as a nurse in caring for people who are dying.

Activity 1.4   Reflection

Think back to the start of your nursing course and reflect on what you thought the role of the nurse might be in caring for someone who is dying. Make a note of these thoughts.

Now think about any time you have been on clinical placement and have seen or cared for someone who is nearing the end of their life. Make a note of your observations and thoughts as to the role of the nurse in caring for someone who is dying in light of these experiences.

Are there differences between your two sets of notes? Did your initial thoughts about what it might be like to care for someone who is dying look similar or different to the experiences you have had?

This is a reflective question, and no answer is provided as this is your own response.

Nurses and nursing are central to both generalist and specialist palliative care provision. Patients requiring palliative care can be encountered anywhere across the healthcare system. The focus of the nurse's role is both the patient requiring palliative care and their family or those close to them. Within this, and reflecting what has been discussed as the focus of palliative and end of life care, nurses support patients and their families with physical, psychological, social and spiritual aspects of their illness. This approach reflects back to Dame Cicely Saunders' original thinking when she adopted the term 'total pain' to describe the complex mix of physical, emotional, social and spiritual elements that people experience at the end of their lives (Saunders, 1996). Within the concept of total pain, the end of life is *as individual as the life that preceded it and that the whole experience of that life is reflected in a patient's dying* (Saunders, 1996, p. 160).

A key component of the role of the nurse in palliative and end of life care is to be 'alongside' the patient and their family, providing presence, actively listening and allowing time and space to explore wishes, concerns, unresolved issues, troubles and to facilitate potential ways of addressing these (Inbadas, 2018). This can perhaps feel like a challenging and overwhelming task to a student nurse who is very new to caring for people at the end of life. It is worth remembering that people who are dying are also people who have lived, who will value the same care, kindness and compassion that you would show any patient. Being with someone and giving them a sense that you are alongside them in their illness can provide a great sense of comfort, of being cared for and of being listened to. Your presence can be a very valuable tool.

The role of nurses in providing palliative care is one that has been evaluated through research, with the aim of trying to systematically establish what it is that nurses see as their unique position in helping those approaching the end of life.

Research summary: The role of the nurse in palliative care

A systematic review of qualitative research conducted by Sekse et al. (2018) aimed to explore how nurses providing palliative care describe their role. They recognised that there

(Continued)

(Continued)

was a need for descriptions of the nurse's role in performing palliative care across all areas of the healthcare system where palliative care occurs.

Sekse et al. (2018) searched for qualitative research papers that had included the following aspects in their research:

- nurses with generalist or specialist palliative care training, or no palliative care training
- nurses who had worked in palliative care for various periods of time
- nurses providing palliative care across different parts of the healthcare system, e.g., acute hospitals, people's homes, care homes etc.

Twenty-eight papers were included in the review which represented the views of 834 nurses providing palliative care in various healthcare settings and institutions. Most nurses worked in hospitals or home care. Eight of the included papers reported research conducted in the UK and nine other countries were represented. The analysis of the papers looked for similar and comparable themes shared between them, as well as identifying aspects that weren't common to each paper; using a process called thematic synthesis (Thomas and Harden, 2008).

The authors of the review identified six key components of a nurse's role when providing palliative care:

1. Being available

   Nurses were the professionals who generally spent the most time alongside patients. The ability to spend time with patients and having frequent and regular contact was felt to enable the development of relationships with patients; these elements facilitated the provision of individualised care for both the patient and their family. Nurses also described themselves as taking on the role of patient advocate; this included ensuring continuity of care where feasible and ensuring that patients understood information and feedback provided to them from other health professionals.

2. Being a coordinator of care for patients and relatives and other health professionals

   Nurses described themselves as the coordinators of a patient's care. Their work was characterised by networking with other professionals and between the patient and their family. Being available and doing what was needed was seen to give nurses a specific and natural role as a hub of other services. Being the professional who undertook liaison and coordination was seen as important for continuity of care, and was achieved through relationship building and good communication.

3. Doing what's needed

   Nurses saw their role as handling an enormous breadth of activities of assessment, planning, intervention and evaluation, of relatively routine tasks alongside highly complex ones.

At the end of life, the 'doing what's needed' was described as providing care that gave comfort to patients through management of physical and psychological symptoms and providing care in the form of bathing, providing mouth care and presence. It was noted however, from those nurses working in more acute healthcare settings that the strong curative culture that prevailed could cause tensions in relation to the value placed on end of life care.

4. Being attentive, present and dedicated

    Nurses said that they were both ambitious and dedicated in their desire to provide high-quality care for people who are dying and their relatives. This also manifested itself in a willingness to carry on working with patients and relatives when relationships were difficult and other agencies sought to withdraw their support. Interpersonal skills and qualities such as kindness, warmth, compassion and genuineness were seen as essential.

5. Being a supporter

    Nurses sought to provide support and education to patients and their families. Caring for the patient's family was seen as a particularly important part of the nurse's role in palliative care and involved making the families feel comfortable and well supported.

6. Lack of time and resources

    Several studies included in the review highlighted the increasing volume and complexity of the nurses' workloads, in addition to limited time for reflection and debriefing. Time constraints were frequently discussed, with the majority of nurses noting the challenges of providing the level and quality of palliative care they aspire to when staffing shortages and conflicting demands on their time minimised the time they had available to support patients. This was a regular source of dissatisfaction for nurses. To counter to this, nurses said how satisfying it was when they were able to provide a level of care which enabled holistic care for patients.

Conclusion of the review

This review highlights how, internationally, nurses perceive their role in providing palliative and end of life care. Given the different healthcare systems and cultures represented across the studies in the review there is a commonality of experience and expectation of the role of the nurse in providing palliative care. There is also a shared understanding of what can cause palliative care provision to be less than ideal.

The review highlighted above has some interesting findings. What it describes as the aspects of care that are fundamental to the nurse's role in palliative care are also those that will be familiar to you as the fundamental aspects of all nursing care. This is an important point of consideration. As the authors of the review conclude:

> *To be able to give individually tailored palliative care to patients with life-threatening illnesses and their relatives, the nurses need all their knowledge of basic nursing. Situations challenge nurses in practical, relational and moral dimensions of care and make demands on their role in a comprehensive way.*
>
> Sekse et al. (2018, p. e21)

An important aspect of this book, therefore, is that the fundamental aspects of the palliative approach to care are relevant to all nursing care, and that the principles of good nursing care also apply within the palliative approach. These elements of care include: seeing a person as an individual, listening to their concerns, placing them at the centre of their care, promoting independence and ensuring that their care is individualised to them. Also important is being alongside them during their period of ill health, and acting as their advocate where this is wanted. You will already have developed skills and knowledge that help you to success in providing good palliative care.

Where do people die and what do they die from?

So far in this chapter we have discussed that palliative care can be provided in most care settings. We have discussed briefly that a palliative approach to care can be applicable in most settings in which people who are living with a life-limiting condition are cared for. What we will now explore is what causes people's deaths and where these deaths happen. Having an understanding of this information will help you start to recognise who may require palliative care and where this care may be required most.

Certification and registration of death data

In the UK we are fortunate to have access to detailed information about what causes people's deaths, how old they are when this happens and where their death occurs. These data are collected through the UK's death certification and registration system and it is a legal requirement to register someone's death after they have died; the timing of this varies between the four UK nations, ranging between five and eight days. Mortality statistics are based on the information recorded when deaths are certified and registered. Most deaths are certified by a medical practitioner either in hospital, at someone's home or in a care home, using the Medical Certificate of Cause of Death (MCCD). This document is commonly referred to as the 'death certificate' and, once completed, it is passed on to someone close to the person who has died, usually a near relative. When a death is registered, details from both the completed death certificate and the person registering the death (the informant) are recorded. These include:

- details provided on the death certificate by the certifying doctor including cause of death and whether a post-mortem occurred;
- details supplied by the informant – for example, occupation of deceased, sex, usual address, date and place of birth, marital status, date of death and place of death.

Once recorded, these data are forwarded to the Office for National Statistics (ONS) by the registrar. The ONS collate all data from death registrations in England and Wales. Similar analyses are undertaken by National Records for Scotland and the Northern Ireland Statistics and Research Agency in these devolved nations.

Causes of death

Taking the ONS data for England and Wales as an example it is possible to determine changes and trends in cause of death, place of death and the numbers of men and women dying; it is also possible to see changes in life expectancy over time. Up to the start of 2020, leading causes of death for men and women were largely unchanged for a number of years and were:

- dementia and Alzheimer's disease;
- ischaemic heart diseases;
- cerebrovascular diseases;
- cancer of the trachea, bronchus and lung.

During the Covid-19 pandemic, Covid-19 became the leading cause of death for both men and women and contributed to an increase in the number of people dying between 2019 and 2020 by 14.5 per cent. Covid-19 led to the greatest number of deaths recorded in any year since 1838, apart from 1918, when the 'Spanish flu' pandemic occurred (ONS, 2021). The lasting impact of these additional deaths on future leading causes of death is not yet known.

It is interesting to note that of the leading causes of death listed above, many of these are not conditions traditionally associated with palliative care. Palliative care services developed in response to the needs of people with cancer at the end of life. Palliative care for people with Alzheimer's disease, dementia and cardiovascular diseases remains an area which is rapidly developing, but is not yet comparable to that for people with cancer.

Where do people die?

A further set of data that can be obtained from death registration information is that of place of death. It is important that we understand where people die as these data help inform policy around end of life care provision, how and where services are provided, or need developing further, and to help target where education and support for healthcare staff is required. Do Activity 1.5 before reading further in this chapter. It asks you to consider where people die.

Activity 1.5   Critical thinking

Rank the following in order from where you think most deaths occur, to least deaths occurring:

Home, hospital, hospice, care home.

An answer is provided at the end of the chapter and discussed in the following section.

The ONS produce five-year averages for 'place of death' data. Table 1.1 details the percentage of people dying in different places between 2015 and 2019. Compare the information in this table to the list you made and reflect on any differences – why did you put the answers in the order that you did? Do the actual answers surprise you?

Hospital is the most common place for people to die, followed by home or care home. In fact, 92 per cent of all deaths occur in these three locations, with only 5.5 per cent of deaths occurring in hospices.

Location of death	Percentage
Hospital	46
Home	24
Care home	22
Hospice	5.5
Elsewhere (outside areas, e.g., beach, mountain, motorway)	2
Other communal establishments (includes hotels, schools, prisons etc.)	0.5

Table 1.1   Place of death 2015–2019 (ONS, 2020)

Where people die will be influenced by a variety of factors. This includes their individual circumstances (such as their illness, symptoms, support needs, whether they have family support, their housing, access to medicines etc.), the availability of care to meet those needs in any given location and their personal preferences.

How can data inform the changing face of palliative and end of life care?

We can learn a lot by looking at data that helps inform us not only of what has happened, but also how we may need to adapt care provision as a result. For example, during the first two years of the pandemic, a shift in place of death occurred with the number of deaths in private homes being almost 40 per cent higher in 2020 compared to the five-year average reported above (O'Donnell et al., 2021). The leading causes of these deaths were dementia and Alzheimer's disease. While the numbers of people who died in care homes and hospitals increased above expected only during the pandemic waves, the numbers of people who died at home remained above expected both during and between the pandemic waves (O'Donnell et al., 2021). The full reason for this increase is not yet known, nor is the quality of care received by the people who died. What is known is that the increase of deaths at home continues and may represent a lasting effect of the pandemic.

These data have implications for planning and organisation of palliative care and community services. There is a sense that we may be seeing the start of a permanent shift in place of care and death, and it may be that more people die at home in the years to come. Already, specialist palliative care providers, such as hospices, have increased their provision of hospice at home services to try and meet this increasing demand. Outreach services are increasingly supporting people who have not traditionally accessed palliative care services, such as those who are homeless, traveller communities and ethnically diverse groups in order that services are adapted to the particular requirements of individual communities, ensuring that everyone who requires palliative and end of life care can receive it.

Chapter summary

In this chapter, we have explored what is meant by palliative and end of life care and considered the role of specialist and generalist care services in supporting people living with life-limiting illness and at the end of life. We have considered the role of hospices, and the pioneering work of Dame Cicely Saunders in developing the modern hospice movement. We discussed the role of nurses in palliative and end of life care, and encouraged you to reflect on your own observation of nursing roles in practice. There is a clear, defined and unique role for nurses to provide patients and their families with high-quality palliative care, and this is relevant to nurses of all fields of practice. Most people die in hospitals, but many people also die in care homes, at home and in hospices. The location where someone receives palliative care and where they die is, to a great extent, dependent on the needs of the individual, but is also influenced by individual preference, the nature of their illness and the availability of services in any one locality.

Activities: brief outline answers

Activity 1.1 Critical thinking (page 10)

Palliative care is not only for people who are expected to die soon. It is for anyone who is facing a life-limiting illness. In some circumstances people may receive palliative care for months or years.

Activity 1.5   Critical thinking (page 20)

Most deaths occur in hospital, followed by home, care home, hospice.

Further reading

Gomes, B (2018) Where is palliative care provided and how is it changing? in Walshe, C, Preston, N and Johnston, B (eds), *Palliative Care Nursing: Principles and Evidence for Practice* (3rd edn). London: Open University Press McGraw-Hill Education, 41–53.

This chapter provides greater detail of where palliative care may be provided, people's preferences around place of death, and some of the changes that are occurring in relation to this.

Useful websites

www.hospiceuk.org/

Hospice UK – this is the website for the charity that supports hospice care across the United Kingdom.

www.mariecurie.org.uk/

Marie Curie – Marie Curie is a charity which provides care, support, information and campaigning for people diagnosed with a terminal illness, their family and those who are bereaved.

www.ons.gov.uk/peoplepopulationandcommunity/birthsdeathsandmarriages/deaths/ methodologies/userguidetomortalitystatisticsjuly2017#information-collected-at-death- registration

Office for National Statistics *User Guide to Mortality Statistics* – This website provides supporting information for mortality statistics, which present figures on deaths registered in England and Wales.

Chapter 2

Person-centred and cultural considerations for care

NMC Future Nurse: Standards of Proficiency for Registered Nurses

This chapter will address the following platforms and proficiencies:

Platform 1: Being an accountable professional

At the point of registration, the registered nurse will be able to:

1.14 provide and promote non-discriminatory, person-centred and sensitive care at all times, reflecting on people's values and beliefs, diverse backgrounds, cultural characteristics, language requirements, needs and preferences, taking account of any need for adjustments

Platform 4: Providing and evaluating care

At the point of registration, the registered nurse will be able to:

4.9 demonstrate the knowledge and skills required to prioritise what is important to people and their families when providing evidence-based person-centred nursing care at end of life including the care of people who are dying, families, the deceased and the bereaved

Annexe B nursing procedures

At the point of registration, the registered nurse will be able to:

10.6 provide care for the deceased person and the bereaved respecting cultural requirements and protocols

Introduction

People with the same health problems may have vastly different priorities for their health care, developed from their differing circumstances, values, preferences and health beliefs. **Person-centred care**, where nurses and other health professionals work collaboratively with people to meet their individual care needs, is fundamental in your nursing practice. In this chapter, we will consider person-centred care and a complementary approach, relationship-centred care, and discuss how these align with the palliative approach to care that we introduced in Chapter 1. We then move on to explore concepts that will help you to understand and explore what is important to people. This includes the concepts of personhood and identity; we will consider how experiencing life-limiting illness will impact on this. We discuss spirituality, exploring how this is sometimes overlooked in nursing care and suggest some ways that spiritual support needs may be assessed in practice. Therapeutic relationships with patients, families and carers underpin any approach to care, and we consider the significance and challenges of developing these. Finally, we will discuss culture, and the impact of this upon people's wishes, values and preferences for care and consider inequity in access to palliative care.

Person-centred care

Students often ask us how they can deliver individualised palliative and end of life care within services that are usually very structured in their routines, processes and procedures. They also want to know how they can get to know a person and what is important to them in a busy healthcare environment when there are multiple competing pressures and demands on a nurse's time and resources. There are no simple solutions to these challenges, but adopting a person-centred approach to your nursing practice will help you to strive to understand the experience and goals of the people who you care for.

'Person-centred care' is a commonly used phrase in nursing. It is one which requires careful consideration to avoid it becoming rhetoric (i.e., organisations and individuals using this phrase, but it lacking in sincerity and meaningful action). Before we start to discuss person-centred care, take a few minutes to do Activity 2.1. This involves you reflecting on your current understanding of what person-centred care means.

Activity 2.1 Critical thinking

1. What does 'person-centred care' mean to you? Write this as a definition starting with the phrase 'Person-centred care is …'.
2. Think of an occasion where you have delivered, or observed care being delivered, to a person at the end of life in a way that you thought was person-centred. Make some notes about why this was person-centred.
3. Critically consider the following question: how do you *know* this care was person-centred?

These are your own thoughts, but we have included some things that you might consider in the outline answers at the end of the chapter.

Person-centred care is hard to define in only a few words, as you may have found when you did Activity 2.1, and there is a lack of clarity across the literature about what this concept means (Öhlén et al, 2017). The NMC (2018) states that person-centred care is *an approach where the person is at the centre of the decision-making processes and the design of their care needs, their nursing care and treatment plan* (p. 39). Activity 2.2 will help you to think critically about this definition.

Activity 2.2 Critical thinking and reflection

Read the NMC definition of person-centred care provided in the previous section and consider the following questions:

1. Does the NMC definition align with your own?
2. Does it fit the example of person-centred care that you identified?
3. What are the limitations of the NMC definition for your practice?

There are no answers provided to this question, as this is based on your own thoughts. We will discuss these issues in the following section.

Activity 2.2 encouraged you to apply the NMC definition to your own practice. The NMC definition emphasises that the person should be at the centre of care in relation to identifying care needs and developing subsequent care and treatment plans. But like most simple definitions that attempt to clarify complex concepts it does not capture the breadth and multifaceted aspects of what person-centred care is. It also does not explain what 'being at the centre of care delivery' means or give any indication of what the best way is to support people to contribute to decision-making. Indeed, supported decision-making is only one way in which person-centred care is enabled; other activities may include self-management support, care planning, partnership working, integrated care, effective communication between patients and professionals and valuing the personhood of patients (Harding et al., 2015). We will explore some of these topics in greater detail later in this chapter.

Price (2019, p. 21) offers a more detailed definition of person-centred care:

> *Person-centred care is a relationship developed with a patient that demonstrates due regard for the personal experience and perceptions of their current situation, which enables people to feel respected, supported and valued during healthcare. It assists the patient to take stock of their circumstances and to explore options for the future, options that may be dependent on what the patient does as well as what is being offered as part of the service. Person-centred care assures the person that we have regard for their wellbeing, a life that has personal meaning, but it also insists on the nurse's role as consultant, expert and advisor, roles that involve sharing evidence, experience and best practice wisdom. Person-centred care is facilitative; it enables the patient to engage and debate to the extent that they feel comfortable, and it always acknowledges their right to informed consent, to accept, augment, to change, to refuse a course of action, whilst also accepting their personal responsibility for the decisions that they make.*

Price's definition highlights fundamental concepts of nursing practice, such as therapeutic relationships, recognition of patient experience and perspective, valuing people and working in partnership with them to plan and deliver care. It recognises the role of the nurse as an expert advisor, but also highlights the rights, autonomy and responsibilities of patients, something that is perhaps less usually considered in relation to person-centred care. Underpinning this are a nurse's effective communication skills which, as we discuss throughout this book, are paramount in the delivery of good palliative care. These issues are important across the lifespan, but arguably are particularly important when working with people at the end of life, when their sense of self can be threatened by living with life-limiting illness. When person-centred care is considered through Price's (2019) definition, the complexity of the approach is demonstrated. It requires significant skill, knowledge and understanding on the part of the nurse to create the conditions in which person-centred care can be achieved.

Limitations of the person-centred approach to care

Person-centred care is widely accepted as an approach to nursing care. However, it does have limitations and is criticised for its emphasis on individual autonomy and subsequently neglecting relational and sociocultural requirements for care (Fang and Tanaka, 2022). The emphasis on individual autonomy is also a dominant western narrative and may lead to people from non-western cultures not having their needs adequately recognised (Fang and Tanaka, 2022). Care for people at the end of life also usually involves a network of people outside the multidisciplinary team, including family members who take on carer roles and other members of the patient's community. Person-centred approaches which only consider the support needs of the patient may overlook the important support needs of these other groups. In Chapter 7 we explore support for carers further.

Relationship-centred care approaches should be considered alongside person-centred care in order to expand the inclusiveness of your practice.

Relationship-centred care

Relationship-centred perspectives offer an additional framework for care and emphasise that the interpersonal relationships that exist in healthcare influence the patient's experience and their health outcomes. Also, that the nature of the relationships that exist in healthcare (between patients and practitioners, between practitioners themselves, and between the community and the practitioner) are significant for enabling health (Soklaridis et al., 2016). A relationship-centred perspective is particularly relevant for palliative care, where psychosocial needs and interventions feature highly in care considerations.

Nurses in some care settings may be involved with someone's care over extended periods of time – for example, in long-term care facilities, such as nursing homes, where deep connections with residents are sometimes developed. Equally, nurses working in community or primary care settings may have known a patient and their family over months and sometimes years. This raises challenges and opportunities for palliative and end of life care. A relationship-centred focus encourages consideration of the needs of patients, families and carers *and* nurses.

Person-centred and relationship-centred approaches are sometimes presented as though care must be either one or the other. In practice, both these approaches (so considering individual needs and the significance of relationships) have value alongside each other.

We will now move on to explore concepts that help to understand what matters to people.

The person in the patient

When someone enters healthcare services, they become 'a patient', a widely used label that relates to their role within healthcare settings. In the following section, we will start to explore concepts that can help you to consider the person, the impact of illness upon their experience and identity, and how seeing the person in the patient (Goodrich and Cornwell, 2008) is the cornerstone of developing effective therapeutic relationships that help people to feel safe, cared about, and which can support people to live well in their circumstances. When a person is identified as approaching the end of their life this can affect their sense of who they are as a person and their relationships with others.

Case study: Luis

Luis had worked hard to support his family and was an active member of his local sports club, where he volunteered as a junior football coach. Luis took pride in being fit and healthy and was looking forward to retirement when he planned to move to Spain to follow a long-held ambition of opening a restaurant with his wife, Greta. Last year Luis had frequently seen his GP as he had pain in his joints, felt tired all the time and started to struggle at work. Initially, the GP suggested that this was due to stress and overdoing it on the football pitch. Greta made him return to the GP when he didn't get better and, following some blood tests, he was invited for a bone marrow biopsy. He later received the devastating diagnosis of acute myeloid leukaemia.

Luis has been speaking with the nurse at the chemotherapy centre about what has been happening. Since his diagnosis and subsequent treatment starting, Luis has been on sick leave from work and has also stopped his volunteer coaching as he has no energy. He is worried about money as he only gets a few weeks' sick-pay from his job. He feels angry that all of their plans for retirement have been for nothing and scared for the future which now seems very bleak. He is struggling to discuss his feelings with Greta and feels very emotional when thinking about what is happening to them.

Personhood

Valuing personhood, or 'what makes you who you are' (Krishna and Yee Kewk, 2015, p. 1) is a central tenet of the palliative approach to care which recognises people as unique individuals with holistic experience and subsequent biopsychosocial support needs. Valuing someone's personhood involves you considering the whole person, which includes their **wellbeing**, their social and cultural context and their preferences, not just focusing on their symptoms or diagnosis (Health Foundation, 2016). Being diagnosed with life-limiting illness can threaten an individual's sense of personhood. People's previous plans and hopes for the future may need to be rewritten, social roles and personal relationships change and the body also changes, no longer behaving in familiar and expected ways. Where a life-limiting illness is **progressive** (i.e., it gets worse over time) physical changes may be permanent and worsening and people experience a series of losses over time. These losses relate to physical functioning, such as changes to mobility, self-care abilities and continence. Additionally, health deterioration leads to numerous psychosocial changes that may also be experienced as loss – for example, having to stop working (often accompanied by financial concerns), giving up a driving licence for medical reasons, being unable to continue with hobbies or leisure activities and experiencing a reduced social network. People may experience changes in their sexuality and sex life which can impact on their relationships. Personal appearance is also often altered through weight loss or gain, changes to hair and skin, or implications of surgical interventions. A person's sense of who they are is challenged and their identity, which arises out of their view of themselves and how others perceive them, may change as illness progresses (Hockley, 2008).

People develop strategies to try and achieve a sense of normality in their everyday lives following diagnosis of life-limiting illness and often want to be treated in the same way as they were before their diagnosis (Fringer et al., 2018). The process of becoming a 'patient' within healthcare and having supportive care needs is a significant transition for many people. People are often very fearful of losing their **autonomy** (their right to make their own decisions), and having personal wishes and needs ignored or overridden can have significant negative impacts for patients, families and people who are bereaved (National Palliative and End of Life Care Partnership, 2021). Advance care planning is a process for supporting people to share their wishes and preferences for end of life care, so that these can be acted upon at a future time if people have lost capacity to make decisions. We will discuss this in Chapter 6.

Activity 2.3 encourages you to apply the theory we have been discussing in this section, to the scenario involving Luis.

Activity 2.3   Critical thinking

Read the case study involving Luis.

1. What things contribute to Luis' personhood?
2. What might impact Luis' identity?

An outline answer is provided at the end of the chapter.

When you undertook Activity 2.3 you will have realised that there are many things that contribute to Luis' personhood, some of which were included in the case study and others that we do not yet know about. For example, it is not explicit in the case study whether Luis is a spiritual person. Spirituality is often hidden as a characteristic but is an important part of many people's identity.

Spirituality

Spirituality is a significant aspect of health and wellbeing and while it is unique for everyone, spiritual needs include living a life with meaning and purpose, experiencing hope, peace, gratitude and love (Marie Curie, 2022c). We described in the previous section the many changes and threats to identity and personhood that people experience when they have a life-limiting illness. People also often experience a loss of meaning and purpose, questioning the core beliefs and values that they had previously held. This leads to spiritual **distress** and contributes to suffering.

Spiritual care is a fundamental component of end of life care. However, it is often overlooked in nursing practice due to lack of understanding of the meaning of the concept, and awareness of how to integrate spiritual care into nursing work (Rogers and Wattis, 2015). There is a vast range of spiritual beliefs and practices, many of which align with established faith systems and religious traditions (Public Health England, 2016). NHS chaplaincy services are a valuable resource to support people with spiritual, religious and pastoral issues (NHS England, 2015).

Exploring spirituality with patients

It is important to consider the spiritual needs of people at the end of life. Using fundamental communication skills, **compassionately engaging** with people in a holistic way that provides them with a sense of meaning and purpose (Rogers and Wattis, 2020) and listening to their stories of their experiences and helping them to find meaning within these (NHS Scotland, 2009) can be powerful tools for spiritual care.

Tools for practice: spiritual assessment

There are several spiritual assessment tools, the HOPE questions are one of these (adapted from Marie Curie (2022c) and Anandarajah and Hight (2001) and summarised below).

These questions can be used to explore spirituality with patients and conversations using these prompts can help people to reflect on what is important to them and identify their sources of support. They can also help to identify needs which can be met through nursing care, and those which may require input from the wider multidisciplinary team.

H: Sources of **H**ope, meaning, comfort peace, strength love and connection

What are your sources of strength, hope and peace?
What sustains you to keep going?
What do you hold onto in difficult times?

O: **O**rganised religion

Are you religious?
How important is this to you?
How does this help you?
Are you part of a religious community?

P: **P**ersonal spirituality practices

Do you have spiritual beliefs that are separate from organised religion? What are these?
What aspects of your spirituality or spiritual practices do you find most useful? Why?

E: **E**ffects on medical care and end of life issues

Has your illness stopped you doing things that give your life meaning and purpose? Are there specific practices we should know about when we care for you?

A link to the full tool is in the 'useful websites' section at the end of the chapter.

Activity 2.4 will help you to explore what spiritual assessment tools are used in your local clinical area and to use these in simulation to develop your nursing skills.

Activity 2.4 Exploring practice and reflection

Find out what tools are used for assessing spirituality in the healthcare organisations that you have placements in. Simulate using these, and the HOPE questions, with a student peer and then reflect on the experience of undertaking spiritual assessment using the NMC reflective account template:

www.nmc.org.uk/revalidation/requirements/written-reflective-accounts/

There are no answers to this activity as it is based on your own reflection.

Recognising spirituality and identifying spiritual distress are important elements of nursing practice, and assessment tools can assist with this. Practising using these tools through simulation, as you did in Activity 2.4, will develop your competence with these. To enable effective use of any tools, therapeutic relationships are needed to develop trust and facilitate the sharing of sensitive personal information between patient and nurse.

Therapeutic relationships

Nowhere is relationship more important than in illness, especially terminal illness. As a human experience, it overwhelms the body, mind and spirit and defines one's existence.

Hawthorne and Yurkovich (2003, p. 262)

Relationships are a fundamental aspect of human life and healthcare is an interpersonal experience. People access healthcare services as they identify a need for assistance with some aspect of their health or are invited to access healthcare through proactive public health programmes such as cancer screening. Healthcare services are delivered by people whose aim it is support people with their health issues. The relationship that exists between service users and nurses (and other healthcare providers) is pivotal in their experiences of healthcare and significantly contributes to how people understand and live with illness. Building a therapeutic relationship is a key aspect of person- and relationship-centred care. This involves activities and interventions that help to get to know people and what is important to them, developing a relationship that enables productive working on an equal level (Ryan, 2022). Effective and empathetic communication is fundamental as part of this and enables you to connect with people.

Tools for practice: communication skills

All nursing care requires good communication. In palliative care effective communication becomes even more significant because of the sensitivity and significance of what is being discussed.

Fundamental skills such as active listening, listening for understanding, clear verbal communication, demonstrating compassion and empathy, non-verbal communication, and provision of appropriate written information are techniques that you will use in your palliative care practice.

To develop your communication skills you should actively engage with any training you are offered as it is through practising these skills that you will become proficient in them. This training may be through your university, or through the healthcare organisations that you have placements with. We will also consider communication in other sections of this book, particularly in relation to the last days of life in Chapter 3, and with families and carers in Chapter 7.

Another way to develop your communication skills is to identify role models who you see demonstrating good communication skills. Observe what it is they do when they communicate with others and work out what skills it is they are using. For example, you could watch their body language, consider the words they use and how they use them and how they are demonstrating that they are listening. You can then start to apply these techniques in your own practice.

As your career progresses and it becomes part of your role to communicate particularly complex or distressing information, you should seek enhanced communication skills training, and support from experienced colleagues (NICE, 2022a).

Recognition that all individuals (both service users and nurses) have different knowledge, skills and expertise that they can contribute underpins the therapeutic relationship. Poor experiences of end of life care are often underscored in some way by a breakdown in relationship between healthcare providers and services users, and ineffective communication.

Box 2.1   Hello my name is ….

In 2013, Dr Kate Grainger, a medical doctor living with incurable cancer, observed that many healthcare staff did not introduce themselves using their name and that this seemingly simple omission was a barrier to human connection between patient and healthcare professional.

Dr Grainger and her husband Chris Pointon established the #hellomynameis campaign to encourage all healthcare workers to introduce themselves by name to patients as the first step towards the development of a therapeutic relationship. The campaign has had significant impact, with organisations from all over the world participating, and has left a lasting legacy for Dr Grainger who died in 2016.

You can read more about this at www.hellomynameis.org.uk/

Considering someone's culture is also important in developing a therapeutic relationship and providing person-centred care.

Culture

Before you start reading this section undertake Activity 2.5 which encourages you to critically consider your own culture.

Activity 2.5   Critical thinking

Think about what you would say to a student colleague about how people from your culture view dying and death, what rituals they participate in and what factors shape this way of thinking and behaving.

To answer this question, you will need to think about what your own culture is. For some people this will feel like a straightforward question, for others this may be more challenging to identify. You may want to read the first paragraph in the following section to help you with this.

There are no answers provided to this activity as these are your own thoughts and experiences.

Culture is a multidimensional social phenomenon that includes the shared beliefs, ideas, assumptions and customs that connect people together. These are expressed through a variety of means such as social behaviours, arts and literature, food and drink, communication and language, shared values and traditions and rituals. Nurses work in multicultural contexts with service users, carers and professional colleagues all potentially being aligned with different cultures.

Having understanding of patients and their families' culture, and being attuned to their values, beliefs and experiences, will help you to support them to adjust to the dying process and improve the quality of your care (Givler et al., 2021). This **cultural competence** involves being sensitive to people's cultural heritage and identity (which includes things like ethnicity, nationality, religion, sexuality and gender) and being responsive to beliefs and conventions that are aligned with this (Care Quality Commission, 2022). This is not simply learning a set of broad cultural principles or practices for different religious or other groups. Nurses should be wary of 'naive culturalism' that draws on cultural stereotypes without consideration of the diversity that exists within cultures and with the individual values that people hold (Six et al., 2020). It is about getting to know about what is important to the person and their family.

End of life rituals and traditions

End of life rituals are an important part of many cultures and are often linked with religious beliefs. This includes rituals involving the dying person, their family and community, rituals involving care of the body after death and burial/funeral rituals. Different religions have differing perspectives about what is important during the final phase of life and what should happen after death and learning about these will give you some context to have conversations with patients, families and their communities about what is important to them at the end of life, although you should never presume what is important to someone based on assumptions about their faith. Rituals and traditions might include having support and involvement from a church community such as in the Church of England (Public Health England, 2016), religious ceremonies or rites that are delivered by a priest to the dying person such as in Roman Catholicism, receiving comfort from hymns, mantras and holy items such as in Hinduism, or not having any religious rites imposed such as in Humanism (Frimley Health and Care, 2021). Some religions may require specific care of the body after death, such as in Islam, where washing and shrouding of the body should ideally be performed by family members of the same gender as the deceased, or the Baha'i faith where a special ring may be placed on the finger before burial (Frimley Health and Care, 2021).

Undertake Activity 2.6 to explore religions that are practised by people living in your healthcare community.

Activity 2.6   Critical thinking and exploring practice

What religions are practised by people who use your local healthcare services?

Use the Public Health England (2016) document *Faith at End of Life: A Resource for Professionals, Providers and Commissioners Working in Communities,* or Frimley Health and

Care (2021) *A Guide to Reaching our Communities in End of Life Care* (see Further reading) to learn more about these religions and their associated rituals.

There are no answers provided to this activity as it is based upon your own reading and local community.

As you will have seen from undertaking Activity 2.6, there are many different beliefs and rituals. People who are affiliated with a religion will have different interpretations of what is important to them about that religion, so you must not assume that because someone professes to be of a particular religion that they follow all of the practices that are associated with that. It is therefore important to know both if the patient aligns their beliefs with any religion and, if so, how they would want that to impact on their care so that appropriate end of life care can be facilitated.

Healthcare in the UK has developed in what is a predominantly Christian country, and many medical practices that have evolved are aligned with Christian beliefs (Choudry et al., 2018) – for example, many hospices are named after Christian saints. This can have implications for people who do not align their religious or cultural practices with this.

Decolonising palliative care

In recent years, international awareness of the impact of colonisation on the development of health systems based on a western medical model and inequalities in health and healthcare for people whose context and culture sit outside of that model has become much greater. Palliative care, while based on an approach which aims to maximise quality of life for all people who face serious and life-limiting illness, is not exempt from critique of the implications of current care models for accessibility and appropriateness of services for all users.

It is widely agreed that the relief of suffering from life-limiting illness through provision of quality palliative care should be a global healthcare priority (WHO, 2021b). However, requirements for the care of people with life-limiting illness will vary depending on geo-political situation, socioeconomic conditions and culture (Ntizimira et al., 2022):

But how do people die who are not fully assimilated to western culture? Consider non-acculturated people throughout Africa and Asia, for example, and indigenous peoples of persistently colonized countries. Are the needs of the dying in Rwanda, Rajasthan, or on the Rose Bud Reservation the same as White middle-class Parisians or Pennsylvanians? Do health and illness, suffering and death, life and after-life, have the same meaning everywhere? These questions are rhetorical, as the clear answer to all is 'no.' For some, wakefulness in the final moments is crucial even if pain must be endured, while others wish to be pain-free even at the cost of alertness. Some want nothing more than to be at home surrounded by family at the end, others want to fight for longer life in the ICU.

Nitizimira et al. (2022)

Palliative care services whose local population includes people from ethnic and culturally diverse groups should be considering the differing meanings that are attached to illness and dying, and how that impacts on the effectiveness of interventions when working with people from diverse communities. Sadly, there is global inequity in access to relief of suffering through palliative care, and the UK is no exception.

Inequity in palliative and end of life care

Equity means to be fair to all people. This is different from equality, which means treating all people equally – that is, the same. In a system that values equality, all people will be offered the same thing, regardless of what their needs are. In a system that values equity, people will be offered assistance based on what their particular needs are to ultimately enable equal access.

To demonstrate this, imagine that you are working with a small group of ten family carers and you have £1000 to distribute to them specifically to help them pay their heating bills. People in the group are from very different socioeconomic backgrounds, and it includes millionaires and people who depend on universal credit. You decide to distribute the money equally to everyone in the group, so everyone gets £100 each. This is an example of equality. While this may seem fair, the millionaire did not need assistance with their heating and the families depending on universal credit still can't pay their bills. An alternative would be to give more money to those who need it most, and no money to those who don't need it for the heating bill. Everyone is treated differently, but the outcome is that they can all pay their bills. Each person's individual needs have been considered and responded to. This is an example of equity.

Unfortunately, there remains significant inequity in access to palliative and end of life care for people from some communities. For example, people with a non-cancer diagnosis, those that live in socioeconomically deprived or rural communities and people over 85 are less likely to access hospice care (Mayland et al., 2022); people from minority ethnic backgrounds are less likely to access palliative care services more generally (Hussain et al., 2021); people from Gypsy, Traveller and Roma communities face many practical barriers to accessing end of life care services and people living with severe mental illness are less likely than others to receive appropriate care at the end of life (NIHR, 2022). This inequity exists as although all people have the same rights to access care in the NHS, consideration is not always given to the particular needs of these individuals and communities in the provision of palliative care services.

Bajwah et al. (2021) undertook research into the response of specialist palliative and hospice care services to people from minority ethnic groups during the pandemic. Their findings highlight some of the issues we have been discussing in this chapter. Their research is summarised below.

Research summary

Bajwah et al. (2021) undertook a cross-sectional online survey of specialist palliative care services response to the Covid-19 pandemic. 277 services responded which included 168 hospice teams.

They found that policies introduced during the pandemic may have had a disproportionately negative impact on people from minority ethnic groups. Five themes were identified:

1. **Disproportionate impact of restricted visiting.** Ethnic groups who would traditionally have large numbers of visitors were unable to undertake cultural and religious prescribed responsibilities such as personal and emotional care and contributions to decision-making.
2. **Compounded communication challenges.** Communication challenges for non-English-speaking patients were exacerbated without family translators, and the use of PPI further hindered communication.
3. **Religious and faith needs at the end of life.** Lack of access to faith leaders, and lack of access to the body after death caused distress as it meant that important rituals, such as the Jewish 'Tahara' and Muslim 'Ghusl' and 'Kafan' where specific procedures are followed to wash and shroud the body while prayers and psalms are recited were not permitted. Some organisations did report close connections with local faith groups.
4. **Mistrust.** A sense that there was mistrust of healthcare services and of interventions such as advance care planning.
5. **Equal service response with a focus on individualised care.** Many services reported treating people equally, focusing on individualised care needs.

The authors recognise that all patients were negatively impacted by the pandemic but suggest that specialist palliative care services that were treating people equally through individualised care were unintentionally treating people inequitably and that people from minority ethnic groups were disadvantaged.

There is still much work to be done to ensure parity of access to palliative and end of life care. However, the inequity is increasingly recognised and the recent *Ambitions for Palliative and End of Life Care: A National Framework for Local Action 2021–2026* (National Palliative and End of Life Care Partnership, 2021) includes the ambition that there is fair access to care for everyone regardless of who they are, where they live or their circumstances.

Chapter summary

Palliative and end of life care principles are closely linked with person-centred and relationship-centred care approaches. Nurses need to consider the impact of illness on a person's identity and their personhood, alongside spiritual needs, and cultural and religious practices. Relationships are a fundamental part of human experience and the development of a therapeutic relationship through activities and interventions that help to get to know what is important to patients, their families and carers will support the delivery of appropriate palliative care.

There is inequity in access to palliative and end of life care which affects people from minority ethnic groups, people with illnesses other than cancer, older people and those that live in socioeconomically deprived communities or rural areas. While there is increasing national attention to this issue, there remains much to be done to ensure parity of access to palliative and end of life care.

Activities: brief outline answers

Activity 2.1   Critical thinking (page 25)

Activity 2.1 asked about how you know that care is person-centred. Person-centred care involves understanding what is important to the person who is receiving care and aligning care with this. Knowing whether care is person-centred or not involves obtaining the views of the person about their care experience and whether they think it is person-centred. This is often overlooked in nursing (and healthcare) practice.

Activity 2.3   Critical thinking (page 29)

Luis' personhood is created by all the things that contribute to who he is. In the scenario given, this includes his values and beliefs, his culture, family relationships, hobbies and employment and hopes for the future.

Luis' identity will be affected by being diagnosed with a life-limiting illness. His current inability to engage with hobbies and employment, his altered vision of the future, his relationship with his wife and family, his needs for healthcare will all be contributing to his experience of living with acute myeloid leukaemia and how he sees himself and how others also see him.

Further reading

Price, B (2019) *Delivering Person-centred Care in Nursing.* Transforming Nursing Practice series. Sage: London.

This book will develop your critical consideration of person-centred care and how this concept underpins your nursing practice. Chapter 8, 'Helping patients and relatives to live amidst dying', is an excellent application of the concept to palliative and end of life care.

Brathwaite, B (ed.) (2023) *Diversity and Cultural Awareness in Nursing Practice, 2nd edition.* Transforming Nursing Practice series. Sage: London.

This text is recommended to extend your knowledge of diversity and cultural awareness.

Doughty, C. (2017) *From Here to Eternity: Travelling the World to Find the Good Death*. London: Weidenfield & Nicolson.

This easy to read, often humorous and fascinating book follows practising mortician Caitlin Doughty as she travels the world exploring death practices and rituals within different cultural traditions.

Frimley Health and Care (2021) *A Guide to Reaching our Communities in End of Life Care*. Available online at: www.eastberkshireccg.nhs.uk/doclink/frimley-community-end-of-life-booklet/eyJ0eXAiOiJKV1QiLCJhbGciOiJIUzI1NiJ9. eyJzdWIiOiJmcmltbGV5LWNvbW11bml0eS1lbmQtb2YtbGlmZS1ib29rbGV0IiwiaWF0IjoxNjM2O TkxNTczLCJleHAiOjE2MzcwNzc5NzN9.G2Ppp2KEPNIUndYyXLvg4P0lacC3i_m5hec5uj1qkG8 (accessed 21 October 2022).

Public Health England (2016) *Faith at the End of Life: A Resource for Professionals, Providers and Commissioners Working in Communities*. London: Public Health England. Available online at: / assets.publishing.service.gov.uk/government/uploads/system/uploads/attachment_data/ file/496231/Faith_at_end_of_life_-_a_resource.pdf (accessed 21 October 2022).

The above two resources are excellent for developing your understanding of different religious and cultural practices at the end of life.

Useful websites

www.youtube.com/watch?v=JPcp58i_5Nw

This short film made by the Open University discusses death rituals around the world.

www.england.nhs.uk/wp-content/uploads/2021/01/Bereavement-Practices-Jan-2021.pdf

These slides, from the National Health and Wellbeing Team (NHS England and NHS Improvement) describe how people with different religious and personal views respond to grief and bereavement. The resource is intended for line managers but contains information useful for all staff working in healthcare.

www.thelancet.com/commissions/value-of-death

This webpage contains a range of resources to explore the story of dying in the 21st century and was published in early 2022 as part of the *Lancet*'s commission into the value of death.

https://meds.queensu.ca/source/spiritassesstool%20FICA.pdf

This webpage links to the HOPE questionnaire, which is a tool for spiritual assessment.

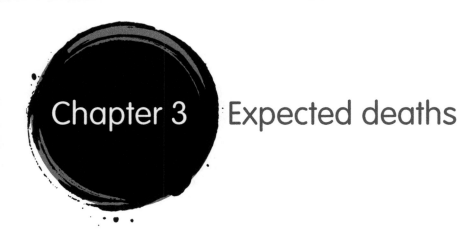

Chapter 3 Expected deaths

NMC Future Nurse: Standards of Proficiency for Registered Nurses

This chapter will address the following platforms and proficiencies:

Platform 1: Being an accountable professional

At the point of registration, the registered nurse will be able to:

1.1 demonstrate the skills and abilities required to support people at all stages of life who are emotionally or physically vulnerable

1.18 demonstrate the knowledge and confidence to contribute effectively and proactively in an interdisciplinary team

Platform 3: Assessing needs and planning care

At the point of registration, the registered nurse will be able to:

3.1 demonstrate and apply knowledge of human development from conception to death when undertaking full and accurate person-centred nursing assessments and developing appropriate care plans

3.14 identify and assess the needs of people and families for care at the end of life, including requirements for palliative care and decision making related to their treatment and care preferences

Annexe B: Nursing procedures

At the point of registration, the registered nurse will be able to:

10.3 assess and review preferences and care priorities of the dying person and their family and carers

Chapter aims

After reading this chapter, you will be able to:

- reflect on your feelings and thoughts about dying and death
- describe common signs that someone is likely to be dying
- understand what is meant by a 'good death'
- give examples of the ways that a student nurse can contribute to care for dying people and their families.

Introduction

Case study: Aran

Aran has recently started his nursing degree. His family are very supportive of his decision to become a nurse but friends have questioned him about how he will feel if he has to look after someone who is dying or if he ever has to look at a dead person's body? Aran brushed this off, but he feels nervous when thinking about death and dying. His great grandparents died when he was a young boy but he doesn't remember a lot about that. When he was in the first year of secondary school, a friend in his class died in an accident. This was an awful time. Aran remembers students and teachers being upset, and some people went to the funeral but he didn't. He still struggles to talk about his friend without feeling emotional.

Aran has his first placement starting in a couple of weeks and he is very anxious that he may be required to look after someone who is dying. Will the nurses think he is no good as he doesn't know what he is doing? What if he says the wrong thing? He's worried too that he might do something to make it worse for the patient or their family, or can't control his own emotions.

Student nurses, like Aran in the case study above, often report feeling anxious about being with someone who is dying or who has died. Many people (including student nurses) will never have spent any time with a dying person. Across your professional career, death will take many forms and your experience of this will vary depending on the clinical settings that you are working in. Some deaths will be because of external trauma such as road traffic accidents, violent crime, or death by suicide. Some will be from internal trauma such as haemorrhage, stroke, or a sudden cardiovascular event.

These deaths from external and internal trauma are generally unexpected. Around 75 per cent of deaths (Royal College of Physicians, 2021) are because of advanced disease or frailty, where there is gradual decline in health. These deaths are expected, can be anticipated and it is these that we will focus on within this chapter.

This chapter will explore what happens during the last days of life. The chapter will start by introducing the idea that despite dying being a normal part of life many people have little actual experience of this. Perceptions of dying and death are likely to be informed by a range of factors which may include personal experience, but are likely to include a variety of media such as film, TV and the news, and you will be encouraged to reflect on the implications of this. This will be followed by consideration of person- and family-centred care in the last days of life. We will consider what is meant by 'death', explore common signs that someone is dying and, critically, consider why recognition of this is an essential component of end of life care. You will be introduced to the concept of the 'good death' and invited to apply this in relation to patient and family carer case studies. We conclude this chapter by considering how, as a student nurse, you can contribute to care during the last days of someone's life and offer some 'top tips' that were developed by our student advisory group.

Dying as a normal part of life

Until relatively recently, death and dying were a common occurrence within families and communities. The rapid rise in medical technology, medication and knowledge that has occurred over the past century means that illnesses that would have been fatal only a few decades ago are now not only curable, but also often considered only a minor problem rather than a life-threatening crisis.

These developments are a positive step and good news in terms of the quality and quantity of life that many people, particularly in affluent populations, get to experience. However, as a result, dying and death have mostly disappeared from public discourse, and daily life. Where death is discussed within the media, this tends to relate to statistics around death; for example, the daily updates of the number of people who had died broadcast during the Covid-19 pandemic, deaths as a result of war or environmental disaster, surprising deaths, such as those of young celebrities, or deaths where healthcare has gone wrong. Rarely is there discussion of deaths that are expected and anticipated.

There are usually around half a million deaths a year in England, and most people will die in hospital or a care home. These deaths will involve only a few people such as close family members and health professionals. As a result, while dying is normal and universal, it is also largely hidden from view. A research survey undertaken in the UK by the Academy of Medical Sciences and Ipsos Mori (2019) identified that most people know little about death and dying, and those that did had learned about this from a variety of sources including personal experience and from friends and family, but also documentaries, film and TV. Activity 3.1 encourages you to consider the implications of this in a little more detail.

Activity 3.1   Critical thinking

Portraying deaths in the media.

1. How are deaths commonly portrayed in the media (e.g., film, newspapers, social media or the news)? Consider some examples of this that you can remember.
2. How many of these are expected deaths at the end of a long illness?
3. What might the implications be for the public who learn about death in this way?

An outline answer to this activity is provided at the end of this chapter.

Activity 3.1 explored how death is portrayed in the media. There are many implications for the public of learning about death in this way, including a lack of awareness about how most people die. The Ipsos Mori (2019) survey also found that people find it difficult to have honest conversations about death and dying. In particular, people would rarely talk about the final days of life and had little understanding of what this might be like. Activity 3.2 encourages you to reflect on your own experiences of talking about dying and death.

Activity 3.2   Reflection

Talking about death and dying.

1. Have you ever had a conversation with someone about the end of life, dying or death?
2. If you have, what did you talk about?
3. How did this make you feel?
4. Was it easy for you or hard for you?
5. What might be some reasons for this?

Make some notes of your answers.

This activity has encouraged you to reflect on your own experience of talking about the end of life, dying and death so no answers are provided. You may find it interesting to repeat this activity when you have finished reading this book to see whether there is any change in your responses.

Care of a person who is dying is a fundamental part of the nursing role and as a student nurse you do not have the choice to avoid talking about death or working with people who are at the end of life. However, we know that many students are particularly anxious about dealing with dying and death. As a result, it takes courage to commit to learning about this. You may have identified this yourself when you undertook Activity 3.2. For some students, learning about death and dying will seem very easy and you will wonder what all the fuss is about. For others, it may be one of the most challenging parts of their nursing education; you may have deep rooted fears about death and dying. It is most likely that you are somewhere between these two extremes. Wherever you are on this spectrum be kind to yourself; recognise that engaging with this material may be emotionally challenging; take a break as needed and talk to your student colleagues and personal and practice supervisors and assessors about your concerns.

The following sections in this chapter will help you to develop your understanding of what happens during the last days of life where death is expected.

Recognising that someone is dying

As we discussed in Chapter 1, someone is deemed to be approaching the end of life when they are in the last twelve months of their lives, but predicting when they will actually die is difficult. Identifying that someone is 'likely to be dying' is a crucial step in creating the conditions for a good death to occur. This enables the opportunity for sensitive and honest conversations to occur with the patient and those that are important to them about their end of life, about what might happen, what support is available and to explore what matters to them during this final period of their life. It also means that patients and families can be involved with care planning and treatment decisions, and that the needs of families and carers can be considered and responded to. Additionally, a plan of care for the last days of life can be agreed and delivered with care and compassion and cultural and personal preferences for care after death can be discussed.

When someone's death is expected, there are often common signs that indicate their death may be imminent. These common signs generally enable clinicians and interdisciplinary teams to recognise when a person may be in the last days of life (these signs are explained in more detail in the section below). This recognition can contain a level of uncertainty and disagreement, and can be more challenging with some illnesses than others (Kennedy et al., 2014). Sometimes it will appear that someone is dying and then they will 'rally' with their condition temporarily improving. In some cases, their condition will stabilise and they will perhaps recover, despite how ill they seemed. Because of this uncertainty, it is preferable to recognise and communicate uncertainty by referring to when someone is 'likely to be dying', or 'is sick enough to die' rather than having a definitive diagnosis of 'dying' (Leadership Alliance for the Care of Dying People, 2014; Mannix, 2018).

Communicating clearly with a patient and their family when dying is likely also gives them the opportunity to undertake any final actions which are important to them such as final conversations with loved ones and religious rites.

The dying person

As a person nears the end of life their body stops functioning effectively, leading to a range of common signs that someone is 'actively' dying, a process that can take several days. These include a range of physical and psychosocial elements:

- **The person may sense that they are dying or have a feeling of impending doom.** They may experience mood and sometimes personality changes alongside social withdrawal.
- **Hydration and nutrition needs will change.** As life nears the end, there may be reduced desire for food and drink and people will eventually stop eating and drinking before they die. Fluid and food should continue to be offered to the patient if they are able and want to take this. Clinically assisted hydration, in the form of a subcutaneous or intravenous drip *may* relieve some symptoms of dehydration but can cause other problems (Kingdon et al., 2021). The decision to use clinically assisted hydration should be taken after individual assessment and in collaboration with the patient and their family (NICE, 2015). Families often ask about nutrition and hydration and, as a student, if you are unsure of the reasons for the approach that is being taken you should seek support from your supervisors so that this can be clearly discussed and communicated with the family. Mouth and lip care should be given every 30–60 minutes to keep the mouth clean and moist – for example, by using ice chips, water sprays/droppers and petroleum jelly on the lips to stop them cracking (NICE, 2021b).
- **Changes to elimination.** Bladder and bowel functioning will both change towards the end of life and support should be given to individuals to sensitively discuss their needs in relation to this so that their dignity can be maintained. As someone approaches the final hours of life they may become incontinent. Absorbent continence pads to absorb the fluid while keeping the skin dry and protected may be a comfortable way to manage this (Marie Curie, 2022a). Constipation and urine retention can both cause discomfort and agitation and should be considered as part of your nursing assessment. Catheters are sometimes used where urine retention is leading to discomfort or agitation, but you should consider that these can also cause discomfort (Marie Curie, 2022a).
- **Reduction in mobility and self-care abilities will lead to increasing need for support with personal care.** This may be distressing for the patient, particularly if this is the first time there has been any need for assistance with personal care.
- **Significant fatigue.** The smallest of actions can feel exhausting and tiredness can occur after only minor exertion.
- **Increased time in bed, asleep.** Gradually, time asleep may become periods of time when unconscious and unrousable. Family and carers may only notice this when they come to wake a person and find that they cannot. A period of fluctuating consciousness, with time awake, asleep and unconscious may last for a few days.
- **Blood pressure decreases.**
- **Agitation and delirium may cause a person to be disoriented and confused.** Sometimes people will have vivid hallucinations and see and talk to people who are not present.

- **Secretions may build up in the chest and throat during the last hours of life.**
  This is because they are not coughing or clearing these in the usual way due
  to being lethargic, asleep, or unconscious. These can make a gurgling, or
  rattling noise; this is sometimes referred to as the 'death rattle'. This can be a
  distressing sound for families and carers but is not generally considered to be
  uncomfortable for the patient. Dr Kathryn Mannix, a palliative care physician
  and author, describes the patient experience of this as being *so relaxed that we
  won't bother to clear our throats, so maybe we'll be breathing in and out through little
  bits of mucus or saliva at the back of our throat. It can make a rattly, funny noise.
  People talk about the death rattle as though it's something terrible, but actually it tells
  me that my patient is so deeply relaxed, so deeply unconscious, that they're not even
  feeling that tickle of saliva as the air bubbles in and out through it from their lungs*
  (BBC, 2018).
- **Breathing patterns change**. There may be Cheyne–Stokes respiration (see the
  Concept summary below for further information about this).
- **The skin will become cool to the touch**. First at the periphery and then more
  centrally. Skin will become more mottled as the circulatory system slows and
  shuts down.

Concept summary: Cheyne–Stokes respiration

Cheyne–Stokes respiration (also referred to as Cheyne–Stokes breathing) was named
after the doctors who identified it in the early 1800s, John Cheyne and William Stokes.
It is characterised by repeated cycles of irregular breathing that is often seen in the
period before death. Shallow breaths increase in depth and speed before halting altogether for a long pause. It is a natural effect of the body's attempt to compensate for
changing carbon dioxide levels. This pattern of breathing can be particularly anxiety-
provoking for families who may be sitting for long periods with the patient. Sharing with
the family that this is a normal part of the dying process and that it does not distress the
patient can provide reassurance.

The dying person may not show all these signs, but when several are present, the fact
that the person may be dying should be considered. Effective symptom management
and good communication with the patient and their family are essential.

All healthcare professionals caring for a dying person also need to be alert to changes
in the patient's status, such as becoming more talkative, having an increased appetite
and changes to energy levels, that may indicate there is some recovery and adjust their
care plans accordingly. This 'rallying' can sometimes last a few hours, but occasionally
last much longer.

Death

Death occurs when there is a cessation of physiological functioning in the body, when there is no sign of cardiac output, respiratory functioning or neurological response.

Care after death

Care given to the deceased immediately following death is sometimes referred to as 'last offices'; however, this term has now largely been replaced with the expression 'care after death', a secular expression which is more appropriate within a multicultural society and which encapsulates a range of activities and processes involving the deceased and their family

Hospice UK (2022) produces detailed guidance on providing care after death. This is a useful and regularly updated resource; we encourage anyone providing care after death to refer to the most recent edition of this. We have drawn on the fourth edition to outline these key principles of care after death, and we include this in the recommended reading for this chapter.

Care after death is an important component of good end of life care. Care shown to the deceased person and their family will have a significant impact on how the family adjusts to life without the deceased. A range of people will provide care to the deceased person and their family from the time of death to burial, cremation or repatriation and beyond. This will include those present at the time of death, those who verify the death, mortuary staff, bereavement support staff, funeral directors, religious leaders, crematoria staff, coroners and many more.

All care that happens after death should be respectful of the individual's religious and cultural wishes and preferences and should aim to preserve their dignity. Clear and compassionate communication with the family is important at all times. When you are first involved with care after death you may find this a difficult process and it may be the first time you have cared for someone who has died. Take the opportunity to ask your nursing colleagues about their experiences of this process and what they do to help them in this activity.

There are legal aspects to care after death and as such it is important that you become familiar with the guidance on this.

Nursing verification of death

Verification of death is a formal process which leads to a record of the official time of death. It can take some time to arrange verification of the death, so families should be made aware that this time will likely be different to the time of the deceased's last breath. In line with all care after death, verification should be carried out with care and compassion, in a timely way that respects the individual, cultural and religious needs of the deceased and their family.

In some circumstances nurses are able to verify expected deaths and Hospice UK (2022a) have published a detailed guide to registered nurse verification of death, which is where we have taken this information from.

Where nurses have been assessed as competent within their care setting they are able to verify adult (age over eighteen) deaths where:

- death has been expected and there are no suspicious circumstances;
- and where a DNACPR conversation occurred between patient and healthcare professional and is documented in the patient's notes;
- and where death has occurred in a private home, hospice, residential or nursing home or hospital;
- where there is no DNACPR conversation documented, and there are signs of irreversible death (rigor mortis) then a nurse can carry out the verification when the other criteria are met.

The nurse who has verified the death also has other responsibilities such as identifying the deceased, starting the process of deactivating any implantable cardiac defibrillators, notifying the funeral director or mortuary where there are any suspected or confirmed infectious diseases or implantable devices (and whether these are still active or not) and informing the doctor of the person's death. They also have the right to refuse to verify a death and to request the responsible doctor attend, or to notify the police if there are suspicious circumstances.

For detailed guidance on the procedure of verification, please refer to the Hospice UK (2022a) *Registered Nurse Verification of Expected Adult Death* (RNVoEAD) guidance which is included in your recommended reading for this chapter.

Communication at the end of life

Effective, timely and compassionate communication with the patient and their family is fundamental in end of life care. While good communication may go largely unnoticed, poor communication can cause significant trauma and distress and, as Dame Cicely Saunders famously said, *how people die remains in the memory of those who live on*. A combination of factors lead to the need for increased attentiveness to communication with patients and families at the end of life. People are experiencing something new in a continually changing situation and may have heightened emotions which impact on their ability to process and retain information. Alongside this they may be being cared for in an unfamiliar environment with unknown routines and healthcare staff they are meeting for the first time. Communicating effectively requires the nurse to listen attentively to what is being said, but also to what is *not* being said, or may be being expressed in other ways. Patients and their families may find it hard to discuss their needs and what they are feeling in the context they find themselves in.

As a student nurse, you may find discussing dying with patients and their families very difficult at first. Take the opportunity as a student to observe how experienced nurses approach difficult conversations including the language that they use, their body language and any other factors that impact on their conversations.

One of the questions that you may particularly dread is 'Am I dying?' (Royal College of Nursing, 2016) or 'Is my relative dying?' When you are asked this, do not rush into a dismissive response, or avoid the question based on your own anxieties. This is often an important opener into a conversation with the patient about what is happening to them. There is no 'correct' way to respond to the question, and the response will depend on the context in which the question is asked. Sometimes using some gentle prompts can help you to understand more about what information that patient is looking for, such as 'Is there a reason you are asking that?', or 'What makes you think that?', or 'Has something happened that has led to you asking that today?' It may be that there isn't a clear answer to the question, or that you do not feel competent or confident yet to have a difficult conversation such as this. In these circumstances you can still play an important role in supporting the patient. Taking time and being with them and actively listening to their concerns, and then finding someone who can explore the question more fully with the person is an important contribution to their care.

Communicating with someone who is dying may sometimes involve you being with them when they are not responding to you, due to their being deeply asleep or unconscious. When providing care in this circumstance, do keep talking to the patient and tell them what you are doing and encourage families to do the same. It is thought that hearing is the last sense to go when someone is dying, so presume that they can hear you and know that you are there with them. Touch is also important. Encouraging families to touch the person or hold their hand or, when they are not there, you sitting with the person and holding their hand is a significant expression of care.

The good death

A 'good death' may seem like a strange expression if you are new to learning about care for people at the end of their lives. Some people may ask 'What could be good about death?'

Let us unpack this a little though; you will start to see that this is a useful concept and that a 'good death' underpins the aspirations of a palliative approach to care.

Although the phrase a 'good death' is widely used across the literature, a more accurate expression might be 'good dying and death' as what it is actually referring to is the period of time around the death including before death, when death is anticipated and death itself. We have already established that death is inevitable and universal, and that people will die in a broad range of circumstances and from a myriad of different causes. Everyone's experiences of death (their own and others) will be different and people will hold different views on what is important to them based on their values, beliefs, experiences, identity, culture and religion, as we discussed in Chapter 2. What constitutes a good death is both socially constructed and fluid. Societies have shared understanding of what factors will contribute to both bad and good deaths. This understanding is not fixed, but has morphed over time and will continue to evolve as culture shapes the way people live their lives, the values they hold and their beliefs about death. Activity 3.3 invites you to consider what matters to you and how that might shape what a good dying or death might look like for you.

Activity 3.3 Reflection

Factors that might make dying better, or worse.

Think forward to the final period of your life when you are dying. What things might make this a more bearable experience? Write your thoughts down. You might want to consider the following:

1. What are the circumstances?
2. Where are you? What is this environment like?
3. Who is there? What is the relationship between these people?
4. What is important to you at this time?

As you continue to read this book, you should consider whether the things that contributed to a better death for you are similar or different to those of other people.

There are no correct answers to this activity, as this will be your own views.

The attributes of a 'good death' are not universal. Your answers to Activity 3.3 will be unique, as will everyone's views of what matters to them at the end of life. What might be considered a good death for one person might be a bad death for another. Research into the concept spans a variety of academic fields including nursing, medicine, health sciences, sociology, philosophy, psychology and thanatology (death studies). The concept is multidimensional and includes biopsychosocial factors linked to quality of life, physical symptoms and symptom management, emotional and psychological wellbeing, spirituality and life having meaning, preparation for death and life completion, and appropriateness of health care (Steinhauser and Tulsky, 2015). The recommended reading for this chapter includes a paper that further explores the concept of a 'good death'.

We will now apply the theory we have been discussing to a case study.

Case study: Elsie

Elsie recently celebrated her 91st birthday. Although she lives with her daughter, Sue, Elsie takes pride in her independence. Her daughter does the shopping and cooking; until recently, Elsie had not required much other assistance aside from using a Zimmer frame to help her walk. Her 90th year had been memorable. It had started with a large party with extended family, including her grandchildren and great grandchildren. She had been on a coach holiday to the Lake District and kept in touch with her large circle of friends through Facebook, some of whom had visited her over the summer.

Over the last few months, however, Elsie had been losing weight and spending more time sat in her chair. She felt like she had less energy to do things and had fallen a couple of times. A serious fall led to an admission to hospital. During her time in hospital Elsie was seen by the elderly care team who asked her lots of questions. They also discussed 'advance care planning', which she found helpful as a prompt to think about the things that were important to her. She agreed that a Do Not Attempt Resuscitation (DNACPR) order should be in place, as, while she enjoyed her life, she did not want invasive medical treatments if her heart was to stop. Elsie valued the frank conversation that the doctor had with her about the success of resuscitation in her circumstances.

Ultimately, Elsie's condition improved and she was discharged home. The community nursing team started to visit regularly, and she enjoyed these visits and got to know the names of the different nurses in the team. If Elsie had any problems, she knew the nurses were coming so could talk to them about this. Over time, Elsie continued to lose weight, had recurrent urinary infections and gradually lost her appetite. She struggled to find the energy to do things that she once enjoyed and needed significantly more help to care for herself, spending increasing amounts of time in bed and asleep. Elsie's GP, in collaboration with the community nursing team, identified that Elsie may be at the end of her life. Elsie requested that she not be admitted to hospital and that she would like to die at home so that she could be near family and her dog, Luna.

Activity 3.4 asks you to apply your understanding of the common signs that someone is dying and of a 'good death' to the case study of Elsie.

Activity 3.4   Decision-making

1. What signs can you identify that Elsie might be sick enough to die?
2. Can you identify any factors that indicate that Elsie may have a 'good death'?

Answers are provided at the end of the chapter.

You may have identified a range of factors in Activity 3.4 that could contribute to Elsie's death being perceived as a good death. Identification of dying, effective management of unpleasant symptoms, accommodating individual's wishes and preferences including for cultural and religious practices and involvement of family and community are important in the provision of palliative care. As with Elsie, this care is delivered by interdisciplinary teams of generalist and specialist healthcare providers working in primary and secondary care settings.

Family perspectives

Family members are those who are likely to care about and have the closest personal connections to the dying person, whether they are formally related or not. Any family's experience of dying, like that of the patient, will be influenced by a host of interrelating factors. These include their relationship with the patient, both over the short and longer term, their knowledge and understanding of death and dying, the role they have taken on in relation to informal care of the person while they have been ill and pre-existing family relationships or tensions. Families may often be anxious about what is happening to their relative as they die and may also be concerned that they receive the best possible care.

Any palliative approach to care should be family-centred. This means considering the needs and experiences of family members both as individuals and as a group. Families can be very diverse and it is important to remember that what you understand as 'family' may be very different to the experience of the people you work with as a nurse. Because of this diversity, it is not appropriate to draw conclusions as to how 'family' experience an expected death, as this will be unique to each family situation and individual members of that family.

The end of a life is a very significant time for families. It heralds a period of transition as the family changes shape and moves to a new form without the presence of the person who has died. Families who are witnessing the end of life period and death of one of their members may be deeply affected by this. Clear and effective communication with families is essential and should include opportunities for members of the family to ask questions and receive comprehensive and clear answers. As a student nurse you should always listen to what a family is saying or asking and if you are uncertain of what the right response is, direct them to someone who can provide this. We provide more information on how to do this in Chapter 7.

Case study: Sue

Sue's mum Elsie is dying and, although she knew this was coming, it feels shocking now it is happening. It had been a challenging few months filled with mixed emotions: periods of deep sorrow as she wrestled with the knowledge that Elsie did not have long to live; fear that she may not be able to care for her; and laughter as she had spent time with her mum going through old photographs, reminiscing and spending time with the extended family.

Over the last few days, Sue noticed a real change in her mum who was increasingly withdrawn, had not been wanting to eat anything and was sleeping more and more. Sue contacted the GP who visited and confirmed that Elsie is likely to be in the last days of her life.

Sue and other members of the family have sat alongside Elsie (whose bed was moved downstairs earlier in the year when she could no longer get upstairs). The community nurses have provided some continence pads as Elsie can't get out of bed any more. Sue could tell that Elsie was really upset when she first used one of these pads. It's the only time Sue had seen her mum really distressed by what was happening to her. The community nurses have set up a small pump which is administering drugs that are keeping Elsie comfortable, and a nurse from Marie Curie has stayed with Elsie overnight so that Sue could get some sleep. The nurse promised to wake Sue if anything changed.

Today Elsie seems different. Yesterday she would occasionally wake up and talk with Sue and other family members, but today Elsie seems very deeply asleep. There is a rattling sound when Elsie breathes, as if she has a terrible chest infection, but the community nurses have told Sue that this is very common at the end of life and that it isn't upsetting to Elsie.

The house is now full of family: her other two children, their spouses and some grandchildren too. The newest member of the family, Elsie's great granddaughter, only eight weeks old, is also there. Family members have taken turns to sit with Elsie, holding her hand, sharing memories of Elsie and family stories, while others have drunk tea in the kitchen. The house feels full of sadness, but there is also a sense of celebration and love. The only time that they leave Elsie is when the carers come to attend to Elsie's personal needs.

As the day has gone on, Elsie's breathing has changed. Occasionally she starts breathing really quickly, and then she stops breathing altogether for a few seconds that feel like much longer. The first time this happened Sue and the family held their breath too. They thought that Elsie had died; it was a shock when she started breathing again, even though the community nurse had explained that this might happen.

This happened a few times, then Sue became aware that her mum had not taken another breath this time. She watched closely, looking for signs that her mum might breathe one final time, watching her chest for its rise and fall, willing her on but also hoping that it was finally over. Finally, there were no more breaths and she knew that her mum had died. She began to cry.

Sue's story is about her feelings and experience of her mum's death. Activity 3.5 encourages you to apply your developing understanding of a good death to this scenario, to consider the significance of communication in Sue's experiences and to reflect on your own feelings.

Activity 3.5   Critical thinking and reflection

1. Can you identify aspects recounted as part of Sue's story that could contribute towards Elsie's death being perceived as a 'good death'?
2. Can you identify examples of where effective communication had impacted on Sue's experiences?
3. How did you feel reading about Sue's experience?

Answers to question 1 and 2 are provided at the end of the chapter. Question 3 is a reflective question and no answer is provided as this is your own response.

As you will have identified by undertaking Activity 3.5, good support for families during the last days of life is an essential component of a palliative approach to care which will live on in the memories of family members, shaping their own perceptions and understanding of dying and death.

Bereavement and grief

When Elsie died, Sue was bereaved. Bereavement occurs when someone who is close to us or important in our lives has died. Grief is our emotional response to the death of that person.

Most people will experience bereavement and grief at some point in their lives. There is no 'right way' to grieve, and everyone grieves differently. Emotional responses include numbness, anger, confusion, relief, feeling overwhelmed, being in shock or disbelief, sadness and depression, and a mixture of emotions. It can affect how people sleep, their appetite, impact on physical health issues and how people interact with others either through withdrawal or wanting to be with others more than usual (MIND, 2022). There is a very broad range of feelings that are associated with grief; these are normal and not a sign of mental ill health. Over time, people usually begin to feel better and start to adapt to their new circumstances, although may still feel periods of intense grief. Sometimes, however, grief may not resolve, and people feel stuck and unable to cope after many months or years. When this occurs it may become a prolonged grief disorder, also known as complicated grief (Cruise, 2022).

Immediately after someone is bereaved they may have a number of practicalities to deal with. This can be a confusing time for people as they experience grief while also needing to navigate procedural and ritualistic aspects of the person's death. These include informing friends and family of the death, obtaining a death certificate, registering the death, planning a funeral and administering the estate of the person who has died (often referred to as 'probate'). If you are supporting recently bereaved families, they may need advice and signposting with 'what next'; hospitals and other care establishments commonly have printed information that can help guide people through this period. People sometimes report feeling abandoned by services and isolated following the death of a loved one, particularly where they have had many people involved with care prior to the death, as Sue had.

There are a lot of voluntary organisations that exist to support people who are bereaved. AtaLoss is a national signposting website that contains details of these organisations, as well as information on emergency support and online bereavement support. Activity 3.6 asks you to look at this website and consider how you might use it to support Sue.

Activity 3.6   Exploring practice and decision-making

- Visit AtaLoss.org and read about what is offered by this organisation.
- Look at the bereavement services page and identify an organisation that might support Sue. For this activity, imagine that Sue lives in your local area.
- Consider how you might use this information to help Sue.

Some suggested answers are provided at the end of the chapter.

In Activity 3.6 you will have explored a range of sources of support for people who have been bereaved. Where people die and the care that they receive during the final period of their lives will impact on their experiences and the grief that families feel after the death. We will move on now to consider locations of care at the end of life.

Locations of care

Where end of life care happens – that is, the location of care – will impact on the experience of patients and families. Hospices are specialist centres of end of life care and are expertly equipped, offering exceptional support to patients and families. Individual homes are familiar spaces, and the preferred location of end of life care for many. However, the adaptations often required during the end of life, such as specialist equipment and daily visits from multiple care providers, can compromise the sanctity of this environment. Hospitals are highly variable spaces; many areas are able to offer a good environment for end of life care, particularly where there is staff expertise, access to private spaces for patients and families and staff/patient ratios that enable individual personalised care.

A patient's preferred place of care (and death) should be ascertained as part of a holistic assessment and can be part of advance care planning, which we discuss further in Chapter 6. People who have undertaken advance care planning may have expressed a preference for where they want to spend their last days of life, although it is important to recognise this preference may change, particularly when symptoms or living situations are unpredictable or unstable. Sometimes the patients and their family may have differing preferences for location of end of life care and supportive conversations and ongoing assessment are needed to resolve these. It is also difficult for people to envisage how the needs of the person who is dying will change and perhaps become more challenging in the last days of life. Even when preferences are clearly stated, it may not be possible to accommodate them – for example, hospice beds are limited and admission is subject to bed availability; end of life care at home is often only possible where family carers are able and willing to provide personal care to the patient between visits from formal carers; people living in residential and nursing homes may not have a choice about the location of their end of life care.

People do move between care settings for a range of reasons during the last days of life. This includes discharge home from hospital settings where this is the patient's preference. In these circumstances, care is transferred to the GP and community nursing teams. There is significant geographic variability in terms of what nursing care is available. Some areas may have specific teams able to support the needs of people who are likely to be dying, other areas may depend on district nurses who are visiting people who are dying alongside a wider caseload of people with varied needs. Equipment such as hospital beds, pressure-relieving mattresses, commodes and hoists can be arranged to support the patient's care at home, although these can take time to arrange and be delivered. Social care (such as carers to assist with personal care needs) can often be arranged at short notice through special funding. Patients may also be transferred into the hospital setting if their needs cannot be managed at home. Dying in hospital is sometimes seen as indicative of a 'bad death', but in many cases hospital is an appropriate care setting where a 'good death' is achievable.

Dying alone

The scenarios of Elsie and Sue have considered a death in a large family, where Elsie lived and died with family around her, but this is not the case for everyone. The Office of National Statistics (2019) suggests around 8 million people live alone, and about half of these people are over the age of 65. This figure is projected to rise further, particularly in older age groups. People living alone who have advanced disease may have specific support needs to facilitate them to remain living independently.

While data can show how many people live alone, we do not know how many people die alone as this information is not routinely recorded. Dying alone may occur when someone dies in their home when on their own, but it may also occur in hospitals and residential facilities when family or staff are not present at the time of death. What it means to die alone has been examined by Caswell and O'Connor (2019). They found that dying alone is sometimes perceived as an example of a 'bad death' and many nurses express a view that people should not be left on their own at the end of life. It has also been acknowledged that for some people, dying alone can be considered to be an example of a good death – for example, where the threat of a loss of autonomy and independence associated with dying means that the patient may have a preference to be alone at the end of life (Caswell and O' Connor, 2019).

It is important not to presume that dying people will want family members present during the last days or hours of life. Anecdotally, it is often reported that a person will die when family members or carers have stepped outside of the room for a few minutes, particularly when they have been holding a bedside vigil. Families should be prepared for this possibility, as it can be traumatic when this occurs and some families may feel that they have failed to support their loved one in this important time.

End of life care plans

Individualised end of life care plans should be developed in partnership with patients, and where appropriate their families, and include specific consideration of food and drink, symptom management and psychosocial and spiritual support needs (National Palliative and End of Life Care Partnership, 2021). Some organisations use standardised templates to support end of life care planning. Activity 3.7 invites you to explore what care plans exist in your local healthcare settings.

Activity 3.7   Exploring practice and communication

Find out whether the organisation hosting your placement uses an end of life care plan template. Request access to look at a copy of this and discuss the document with your practice assessor or supervisor, considering when and how this is used.

There are no answers provided as this activity is based on your conversations in the practice setting.

The care plans that you found by undertaking Activity 3.7 may have incorporated guidance that prompts the clinical team to consider a range of interventions that may be helpful for the patient and their family. Any template used for care planning must never replace your clinical judgement.

Being a student nurse and contributing to care in the last days of life

As a student nurse you can make an important contribution to care in the last days of life, even while you are developing your competence and confidence. While you observe the practice of experienced colleagues, offer to participate in any care activities and take opportunities to spend time with patients, their families and all members of the interdisciplinary team. Do not underestimate the importance of seemingly simple interventions. Making some tea for family members, sitting with a patient when they are on their own, asking how someone is today and meaning it, and listening to the stories that people share are examples of important aspects of care delivery that you can undertake. Humans are storytellers, we thrive when we have the opportunity to recount important elements of our lives and you can pay witness to this through active listening and your compassionate presence. It is important also to consider the impact on yourself of caring for someone at the end of their life; self-care is vital in these circumstances and throughout your nursing career. We talk more about self-care in Chapter 5.

Box 3.1   Student top tips

These 'top tips' for working with patients and families in the last days of life were suggested by our student advisory group.

1. **It is OK to cry.**

    Sometimes it is OK to cry with families; dying can be sad and it can be helpful to show that you have a human response.

2. **Death can be noisy!**

    Noises from the patient as they die, and the family as they express their emotions, can be unexpected and surprising.

3. **Ask the family how they are.**

    Families will often want to talk to you but may be concerned about taking your time. Show them that you have time to talk with them.

4. **Ask to see a picture of the patient when they were well.**

    Talk to the family about this and good memories they have. Communicating with families is an extension of caring for the patient.

5. **Talk to the nurses you work with about their tips for caring for dying people and their families**. Nurses will have lots of experience and will usually be very pleased to share this with you.

Chapter summary

This chapter has framed dying as a normal, yet often unfamiliar, part of life and suggested that the ways in which people learn about dying will inform their perceptions and understanding of the final days of life. You have explored the common signs that someone is dying and the significance of good communication. Activities included in this chapter have encouraged you to reflect on your feelings about learning about dying, to apply your knowledge to case studies and to critically consider factors which may contribute to a good death. Finally, the chapter has explored the important contribution that you can make as a student nurse to the care of people who are dying and their families.

Activities: brief outline answers

Activity 3.1   Critical thinking (page 43)

When considering this answer, you may have thought about examples from the news, in films or on TV, or from your social media accounts.

It is likely that very few of these deaths were expected deaths. Most deaths presented within the media are traumatic deaths that can be sensationalised in some way (such as traumatic deaths and celebrity deaths).

The media has a significant impact on how the public learns about health and illness. Representations of dying and death within the media (such as on films, television, in the news and on social media) shape how the public understands what dying is and how this happens. An under-representation of dying as a normal occurrence at the end of a life, and lack of discussion of what this is like lead to a lack of public understanding of common experiences at the end of life. This has implications for how death and dying is discussed within society, and for how people understand dying in relation to their own and others' lives.

Activity 3.4   Decision-making (page 51)

1.   The following (when taken together) are signs that Elsie might be dying:

- advanced frailty
- exacerbation of falling
- weight loss
- recurrent infections
- lack of appetite
- increasing care needs
- reduction in energy
- sleeping more.

2.   The following factors may contribute to Elsie having a good death:

- Elsie dying at the end of a long life, with a short period of disability
- advance care planning conversations with the healthcare team
- open discussion of DNACPR while in hospital
- good relationships with the healthcare team which enable Elsie to discuss any issues or concerns she has
- clear communication with Elsie that she is likely to be dying
- Elsie dying in her preferred place of care.

Activity 3.5   Critical thinking and reflection (page 54)

1.   There are a few elements of Sue's story that may contribute to Elsie having a 'good death', including:

- Elsie having the opportunity during her final months to reflect on her life, and to share this with family
- Elsie dying in her preferred place of care
- family being present during Elsie's final days as per her wish
- effective symptom management

- family being prepared for what happens during the last days of life and having support from the interdisciplinary team with this.

2. Good communion featured several times in the scenario. This included:

- the GP communicated that Elsie was likely to be in the last days of life
- the Marie Curie nurse agreeing to wake Sue if Elsie's health changed. This is often very reassuring for families and allows them to rest for a while
- the community nurses telling Sue about what it may be like as Elsie dies, including the noises that she may make while she is breathing, and about Cheyne–Stokes (the pattern of stopping and starting) breathing.

Activity 3.6 Exploring practice and decision-making (page 55)

AtaLoss.org contains a broad range of services that may be able to support Sue. There are two ways that you could use this website to support her. You could let her know about the website, writing down the web address for her, so that she could access this information herself. Alternatively, you could look at the website and identify specific services that may support Sue, depending on her needs at that point, and give her the information about these. General Practice is also a good place to seek support when bereaved.

Further reading

Mannix, K (2017) *With the End in Mind: How to Live and Die Well.* London: HarperCollins.

This book contains numbers of short stories that explore the process and experience of dying.

Krikorian, A, Maldonado, C and Pastrana, T (2020) Patient's perspective on the notion of a good death: a systematic review of the literature. *Journal of Pain and Symptom Management,* 59(1), 152–164.

A systematic review which explores patient perspectives on a 'good death'.

Hospice UK (2022) *Care After Death* (4th edn). London: Hospice UK.

Detailed guidance on good practice for care after death. Pages 24–30 include information on personal care after death.

Hospice UK (2022a) *Registered Nurse Verification of Expected Adult Death (RNVoEAD) Guidance* (5th edn). London: Hospice UK.

Detailed guidance on registered nurse verification of death.

Annotated list of useful websites

www.mariecurie.org.uk/professionals

This website provides useful information for clinical professionals working with people at the end of life.

www.bbc.co.uk/ideas/playlists/dying-thoughts

This BBC collection contains short films that discuss a range of issues around dying.

www.nice.org.uk/guidance/ng31

This website contains the NICE guideline for the *Care of Dying Adults in the Last Days of Life.*

www.AtaLoss.org

A comprehensive signposting website to sources of support for people who are bereaved.

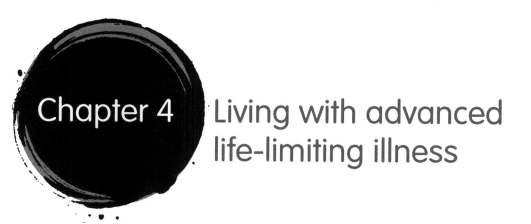

Chapter 4 Living with advanced life-limiting illness

Chapter aims

After reading this chapter, you will be able to:

- identify challenges to health for people with advanced life-limiting illness
- discuss factors which contribute to living well
- describe the rehabilitative approach to palliative care
- critically consider the role of symptom management as part of a palliative approach to care.

Case study: Rosa

Rosa was terrified when she was first told that she had advanced breast cancer. She was scared of dying and desperately sad that she probably would not see her children grow up, and that her wife would become a widow. She was also afraid of what it meant to live with a terminal illness. Would she have to give up the job that she loved? What about her hobbies? Could she still be a good mum? Would she be dependent on other people and lose her independence, autonomy and dignity? She did not know how she could live with the uncertainty of not knowing how much time she had left or what that might be like.

Introduction

Diagnosis of a life-limiting illness can be a shocking interruption to an envisaged future life and to an individual's wellbeing. Like Rosa in the case study above, most people who are diagnosed with a life-limiting illness will experience feelings of fear and uncertainty about what will happen to them and what their life will now be like. Mitchell (2018) has written about living with dementia and discusses that this experience has a beginning (noticing symptoms and receiving diagnosis), a middle (living as best you can in the circumstances you are in) and an end (dying and death) and this same principle applies to all life-limiting illnesses, although the timescales involved will be different. Rosa is in the 'middle' stage of living with her illness, and it is this stage that is our focus here.

Advances in medicine have meant that many incurable illnesses can now be managed effectively for long periods of time, and having a life-limiting illness does not preclude people from living well, or having positive wellbeing. Living well and having good wellbeing are fundamental elements of living a good life and experiencing contentment and happiness; they are ultimately what enable people to thrive. The promotion of wellbeing is increasingly seen in health policy and initiatives, where 'health and wellbeing' are referred to alongside each other reflecting a holistic vision of care where feeling good is a valued outcome.

This chapter introduces you to the idea of living well with life-limiting illness and explores ways to achieve this. We will start by considering the physical changes that people with life-limiting illness face. First, we discuss what 'health' means in this context and describe three common trajectories of illness: a terminal illness trajectory; a chronic disease trajectory; and a dwindling trajectory, one seen more frequently in people with frailty and dementia. We will move on to look at how changes over time impact upon a person's functioning and on their sense of dignity and quality of life. Having established that life-limiting illness can be experienced in terms of a time of change, and of loss, we will introduce you to the rehabilitative approach to palliative care. This approach focuses on working towards goals that are important to an individual and promoting autonomy, choice, dignity and independence. Finally, we will consider the importance of symptom management to living well.

Health and life-limiting illness

When someone is diagnosed with a life-limiting illness, it is the start of a new phase of their life and people often have questions and concerns about what will happen to them, just as Rosa had in the scenario at the start of this chapter. To understand what will happen to someone over the course of their illness, we need to consider what 'health' is and how health might change.

As a student nurse, the core of your role relates to health; you will be familiar with this important concept for which definitions vary depending on cultural and historical perspectives. In writing this book, we have taken a biopsychosocial-spiritual understanding of health.

An **holistic** biopsychosocial perspective recognises the interplay between biological, psychological and social factors on health and health outcomes. Spiritual factors are also important (as we discussed in Chapter 2), particularly in relation to end of life care, which is often a time of ritual and reflection; some versions of the biopsychosocial model also include an additional spiritual element. Table 4.1 highlights some factors which will contribute to health and wellbeing for people with life-limiting illness.

Biological	**Psychological**	**Social**	**Spiritual**
Age	Attitudes	Socioeconomic status	Spiritual beliefs
Genetics	Past experiences	Family dynamics	Religious beliefs
Pathophysiology of disease	Coping	Employment	Faith
Drug effects	behaviours	Social and community networks	
Comorbidities	Emotions	Education	
		Environment	

Table 4.1 Factors contributing to health and wellbeing in life-limiting illness

Health and wellbeing exist on a continuum, and there are usually areas of everyone's lives where their health and wellbeing could be improved. The range of factors that influence health and wellbeing help to explain why everyone's experience of living with illness is unique. Despite this uniqueness, there are commonly experienced and observed patterns of change over time. Different types of disease cause different typical patterns of change and these are referred to as a disease trajectory.

Disease trajectories

Disease trajectories are a way of depicting typical patterns of change over time in different patient groups. They have been used in the medical and nursing literature since the 1990s. Trajectories are presented as simple visual diagrams. In these diagrams, time is shown on the bottom axis, with function on the side axis and as you study these diagrams you will notice that each has a different pattern over time towards very low functioning and death. We will explore three of these trajectories drawing on influential work by Lynn and Adamson (2003) and Murray et al., (2005) where the models are applied to palliative care; the terminal illness trajectory, the chronic illness trajectory and the dwindling trajectory.

Terminal illness trajectory

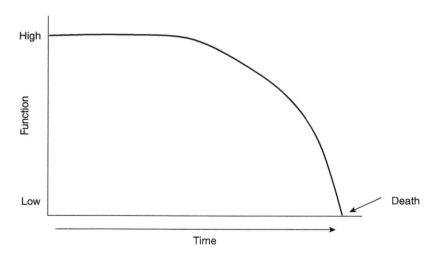

Figure 4.1 The terminal illness trajectory

The terminal illness trajectory includes incurable conditions with a generally predictable progression, such as some cancers. The typical trajectory of a 'terminal' illness is presented as starting from a high level of functioning which may be maintained for years until near death, where there is a steep and life-limiting decline which may occur over a period of months, although sometimes less. We have used the phrase 'terminal illness' as this is reflected in the literature; however, we suggest that it is a phrase that should be used cautiously in your clinical practice with patients and their families. 'Terminal' means the end of something – in this case the end of life. Patients and families can interpret this as meaning that nothing else can be done for them which is not the case as a palliative approach to their care should continue. This may include active treatments that aim to prolong life and should include interventions to help manage symptoms and which promote psychosocial health and wellbeing.

Concept summary: cancer

'Cancer' is a word that often has strong connotations with suffering and death and can be a particularly frightening possibility and diagnosis for patients. There are over 200 types of cancer and there is significant variation in **aetiology**, symptoms, treatments and survival rates. Outcomes for patients will be affected by a range of factors such as stage of diagnosis, other comorbidities and access to services. For the 27 most common cancers, average five-year survival rates in England are lowest for mesothelioma (7.2 per cent), pancreatic cancer (7.3 per cent) and brain cancer (12.8 per cent) and highest for testicular cancer (97 per cent), melanoma of skin (92.3 per cent) and prostate cancer (88 per cent) (Nuffield Trust, 2021). The variability in survival rates and approaches to treatment can be confusing for the public and careful communication is required when discussing cancer.

Chronic disease trajectory

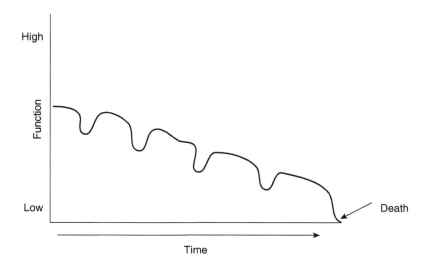

Figure 4.2   The chronic disease trajectory

The trajectory of chronic disease is presented as starting with a moderate level of functioning, followed by gradual decline, with significant troughs which represent exacerbations of illness. These exacerbations may require additional nursing and medical intervention or hospital admission to manage, and from which previous function is not usually fully recovered. This pattern may last for several years and applies to diseases such as chronic obstructive pulmonary disease (COPD) and heart failure. In this unpredictable pattern of progression, death may appear to have occurred without warning, as the exacerbation mirrors what has happened previously from which the person has recovered most of their previous functioning.

The dwindling trajectory

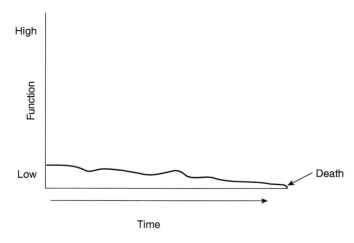

Figure 4.3   The dwindling trajectory

The dwindling trajectory applies in those circumstances where the cause of deterioration in health isn't due to terminal or chronic illnesses, such as in case of frailty or dementia, and often occurs in older people. The trajectory is presented as starting from a fairly low level of functioning, which then has small dips and improvements in a dwindling approach towards death. This trajectory can last several years, and death can often be hard to predict due to the modest fluctuations in health that are occurring. Death for people with frailty and/or dementia often occurs due to other causes, such as an infection.

Concept summary: frailty

Frailty is an abnormal health syndrome that occurs due to decline in reserves across different physiological systems which then impacts on functioning through a range of health deficits (including effects on physical ability, cognitive function, wellbeing and energy). Frailty is increasingly present in older age (although it is not inevitable), rising from a prevalence of 5 per cent of people aged 60–69, to over 65 per cent of people over 90 (NIHR, 2017).

Most people with frailty will also have multimorbidity. Evidence suggests that frailty may be reversed, or progression slowed, through interventions that aim to develop strength and muscle mass and increasing intake of protein (Travers et al., 2019). Older people may not understand how the term 'frailty' is used in medical context, and infer that this relates to them being fragile. It can as such be perceived by older people to have negative connotations. This may impact on how they engage with care or services targeted at people with frailty, and nurses should consider the language they use in relation to this.

In the following case study, these three trajectories are illustrated using the experiences of Jacob, Rita and Marc.

Case study: Jacob, Rita and Marc

Jacob, Rita and Marc are residents of The Grange residential home. Jacob has previously been identified as having severe frailty and currently has a urine infection: he has been mainly in bed for the last two years and has needed lots of assistance with all activities of daily living. Jacob's physical health has declined slowly and there have been times before when the nurses thought that Jacob might be dying, but each time he has rallied. Rita has advanced COPD: over the past twelve months she has had several acute exacerbations of her condition where she experienced a range of unpleasant symptoms including marked increase in breathlessness and tachypnea, peripheral oedema, was observed to be 'purse lipped breathing', had a significant reduction in her self-care abilities and was admitted to hospital. When returning to The Grange, the carers have noticed that she is not able to do all the things that she could before the exacerbation and needs more help. Marc has incurable lung cancer: he had been fairly active around the home until a few weeks ago and the carers have noticed that he is needing much more help with personal care needs, and is unusually fatigued, preferring to stay in bed sleeping for most of the day.

In Activity 4.1, you will apply your knowledge about illness trajectories to the case study of Jacob, Rita and Marc.

Activity 4.1 Critical thinking and communication

Imagine you are on placement with the district nurses and have today visited The Grange residential home. The staff have expressed their concern about Jacob, Rita and Marc and their changing care needs, and wonder whether this is a sign that they may be dying.

(Continued)

(Continued)

Using the three trajectory models consider the following questions.

1. How might you use the trajectory models for explaining the changing health and support needs of Jacob, Rita and Marc?
2. What are the limitations of using the trajectory models to understand what is happening with Jacob, Rita and Marc's health?

No answers are provided for this activity as this is based on your own thoughts, but we will explore these issues in the following section.

Understanding the typical trajectories of different conditions can be useful as explored in Activity 4.1. As Murray et al. (2005) suggest, when people ask about prognosis (like the carers in The Grange), they are rarely simply asking about how long there is left, but also asking about what that time might be like. In referring to the trajectory models with care home staff, you could have explained what a typical trajectory of functional deterioration might look like. This would help to explain that for people with frailty like Jacob, it can be difficult to predict when death might occur and whether a deterioration in health is an indicator of this. It can also help to develop their understanding that it is not uncommon for people in Rita's situation to not fully recover after serious exacerbations, and that Marc's recent deterioration may be an indicator that he is approaching the final phase of his life. This in turn might help The Grange to plan for the possible changing care needs of their residents over time. For all the residents, advance care planning would be appropriate; this is discussed in Chapter 6.

The trajectory models presented do have limitations, as they are very generic approaches. We have described here three commonly presented trajectories, but there are a huge range of illnesses that will result in death encompassed within these. These illnesses have their own nuanced typical symptoms, treatments and types of service provision, all of which will impact on the course of the illness. People with **multimorbidity** and who have illnesses that link to several different typical trajectories may find that these models do not relate to their individual circumstances. When applying these models to Jacob, Rita and Marc's situation, it is most important that their unique situation is considered and reversible causes of the change in health are identified and, if appropriate, addressed. Nursing care should be based on the experience of the person you are caring for when applying theory within person-centred care delivery.

In the trajectory diagrams the 'dips' that occur in each of the lines over time represent a reduction in individual functioning. We will explore what this means in the following sections.

Functional changes

Looking at the trajectory diagrams gives some indication of common patterns of change in life-limiting illness. What they do not tell us is what types of change people are experiencing and how these impact on their daily life. These were the fears that Rosa was voicing in the case study at the beginning of the chapter.

When we consider 'function' we are discussing the individual's abilities to undertake the activities that enable them to live or, to put it another way, how they function in everyday life. This includes how they take care of themselves (such as maintaining nutrition through shopping and food preparation and personal hygiene needs such as washing and dressing), their performing of usual roles within their family, workspace and community, and how they maintain their health and wellbeing (Sargent, 2017). Activity 4.2 will encourage you to reflect on the experience of illness on functioning.

Activity 4.2   Reflection and critical thinking

Consider a time when you have been unwell with a minor illness.

- How did this impact on your functioning?
- What were the short-term implications of this?
- Were there any longer-term implications?
- Refer back to Figure 4.1. Were there any aspects of your biopsychosocial health that you could have altered to improve your health and wellbeing?

There are no answers provided to these questions as these are based on your own experience, but we will discuss this in the following section.

When you undertook Activity 4.2 you may have identified a range of temporary changes to your functioning, such as not getting out of bed for a few days, not wanting to eat or not being bothered to cook or go to the shops. You may have taken a few days off from placement, study, or a part-time job and not met up with friends or work colleagues and felt a little isolated. You may also have family responsibilities or children to care for and may have needed someone else to help with this. Hopefully, these impacts on your functioning were short-lived but there may have been longer implications for you, such as not doing as well in an exam as you had lost time to prepare, or losing income due to not attending part-time work and having to borrow some money to pay bills.

In a life-limiting, longer-term illness the implications for functioning will be more significant. A person's functioning will change over the course of their illness with declines occurring due to disease progression, unmanaged symptoms of disease and treatment, and coping. Some deterioration may be reversible – for example, chemotherapy side effects may mean that during treatment a person experiences symptoms such as fatigue and nausea and struggles to cope, so takes time away from their employment or may need additional support with caring for children. Once treatment has concluded and symptoms are resolved they may be able to return to work and resume childcare. Some deterioration may be longer lasting or permanent and qualitative research of people's experiences of living with life-limiting illness often identifies this as being a series of losses across the biopsychosocial-spiritual domains.

When functioning changes due to illness, you need to consider that a person's sense of dignity can be threatened.

Dignity

Living a life with dignity is important to most people. Dignity is not a simple concept to define but relates to the rights of an individual to be treated with respect in relation to their beliefs and values. The maintenance of dignity is an essential component of care, and reflects the holistic, person-centred focus of nursing practice. Treating patients with dignity and respect are part of the Future Nurse Standards (2018) and also mandated in the UK Health and Social Care Act 2008 (Regulated Activities) Regulations 2014 which are overseen by the Care Quality Commission (gov.uk, 2014).

Activity 4.3 encourages you to reflect on the concept of dignity and to apply this to practice.

Activity 4.3   Reflection and application to practice

Reflect on the following questions.

1.   What does dignity mean to you?
2.   In what circumstances might someone with a life-limiting illness feel that their dignity is threatened?
3.   What actions have you taken as a student nurse to preserve the dignity of a patient? Think of specific examples.

No answers are provided to this activity as it is based on your own views and nursing practice. We will discuss these issues further in the following section.

You may have identified in Activity 4.3 that a declining ability to undertake usual activities and increasing requirements for assistance are significant transitions in life that may threaten an individual's feelings of dignity. People are often concerned about being a burden to their family and to professional support networks and fear the loss of autonomy and independence that will result from their illness. Experiencing increasing dependency can impact a person's sense of identity – their experience of who they are as a person and their sense of control over their own life (which we discussed in Chapter 2). These factors contribute to a loss of sense of dignity.

Research summary

Rodríguez-Pratt et al. (2016) undertook a systematic review to explore the relationship between perceived dignity, autonomy and control at the end of life. They included 21 studies which involved in total over 400 participants. They identified a range of issues that impact on the loss of sense of dignity, including loss of bodily function, changing ability to undertake activities of daily living, altered body image, quality of life and self-esteem, loss of self and self-worth, altered roles, fear of being vulnerable, fear of suffering, control over the body and control over death, rights to choose and decision-making. They found that sense of dignity is further shaped by the illness, the social context and the personal identity held by the patient.

Promoting and maintaining personal dignity is an essential component of nursing practice and is linked to a person's quality of life.

Quality of life

There are a broad range of definitions of health-related quality of life, which is generally understood to be the subjective experience of individuals in relation to their circumstances about how satisfactory, or not, their life is. This umbrella concept includes domains related to physical health (e.g., pain and fatigue), psychological factors (e.g., self-esteem, feelings of positivity or negativity), independence (e.g., ability to perform activities of daily living, capacity for work), social relationships (e.g., personal relationships, support networks and sexual relationship), environment (e.g., availability of care services, home environment, financial resources) and spiritual and personal beliefs (e.g., meaning and purpose in life) (Skevington and Bönke, 2018). Quality of life surveys are sometimes used as a measure of the effectiveness of interventions in palliative care research and practice.

Living with life-limiting illness does not mean that a person will automatically have a poor quality of life. Physical health is considered to be only one component of quality of life, and a person may have challenges in relation to physical health, but strengths in relation to other domains. Quality of life and wellbeing are closely linked concepts and are sometimes used interchangeably. The palliative approach to care places considerable focus on improving quality of life as an outcome of care interventions that help people to live with their illness.

Supporting people to live well with life-limiting illness

So far in this chapter we have explored a range of physical and psychosocial implications of living with life-limiting illness and highlighted that this is often depicted in terms of living with a series of losses for which increasing support will be required to meet individual needs. This way of thinking about advanced illness can be focused on deficits and dependency. In the following sections we explore ways to support people to 'live as well as they can in their circumstances' that promote autonomy and choice and maximise independence.

The rehabilitative model of palliative care

All palliative care focuses on quality of life, and the rehabilitative model of palliative care offers a framework to work towards this. As Tiberini and Richardson (2015) describe, the rehabilitative model is a relatively recent development in palliative care. It is a person-centred integrative model of both rehabilitation and palliative care that works to actively improve people's quality of life by optimising their ability to function within their world through focused support which aims to meet their personal goals and priorities. This empowers patients and families to manage their circumstance with greater independence and with autonomy, choice and dignity.

Within the rehabilitative model, it is presumed that the person (and their family) would like to choose if they want or need support as autonomous individuals. They are viewed as active partners in care and are enabled to make choices in relation to participating, or not, in this. They are partners in care and therefore care is delivered 'alongside them', rather than 'to them' and the focus of care will align with the person's own goals and preferences, rather than the professionals' needs to care for them, or their views on what is best for them (Tiberini and Richardson, 2015).

Person-centred goal-setting and the promotion of functioning (including through symptom management) are important mechanisms for care in the rehabilitative model. We will explore these more in the following sections.

Person-centred goal-setting

Case study: Rosa (continued)

Rosa had been thinking about her future. She knew that her condition was incurable, and that it was unlikely that she would see her children grow to become adults. What she really hoped was that she would live to see her children starting school, so that they might have some memory of sharing such an important milestone in their lives with her. This seemed such a long way off though, as her children were so young at only three years old and eighteen months old. At the moment all her thoughts were focused on her illness and it was difficult to see beyond that. She was particularly troubled by a niggling pain in her hip that was making her irritable and making it difficult to pick the children up or to play with them. If only she could get on top of this pain!

Everyone has things that are important to them, which they hope to achieve and that give their life meaning and purpose. These are underpinned by values, beliefs, wishes and preferences. When patients are asked to consider their wishes and preferences in relation to future care (such as locations of care when they are dying and who they might want to make decisions for them if they lose capacity to do this for themselves) this is referred to as advance care planning, and we discuss this further in Chapter 6. When healthcare professionals and patients work together to establish what matters to the patient, and how current care plans and interventions can be aligned with this, the process is referred to as goal-setting (or goals of care) and that is what we discuss in this section. In Activity 4.4, you will consider Rosa's situation and what goals might be important to her.

Activity 4.4   Critical thinking

Re-read the case studies involving Rosa from the beginning of this chapter and this section.

From these scenarios, what do you think matters to Rosa that might inform goal-setting conversations?

An outline answer is provided at the end of the chapter.

In Activity 4.4 you may have identified a variety of factors from what you know about Rosa's situation, such as her desire to pick her children up and to play with them. In care situations, you would ask the person what matters to them, using your communication skills to help explore this. During the course of an illness, people are required to make decisions about interventions to help them manage their condition and in doing so may need to consider what it is they hope to achieve. Understanding a person's goals for current and future care can help you to support them in making these decisions. These will vary from seemingly very significant decisions – for example, whether to continue to pursue a possible life-extending treatment despite significant side effects – to seemingly more routine decisions, such as which route of administration of medication might suit them best, or what would improve their quality of life while a hospital inpatient. Patients and healthcare professionals may have differing views as to what the best course of action is, so establishing what is important to the patient and what matters to them is important as part of person-centred care.

A goal-setting approach to care may improve patient involvement in their own care. This can occur through improved partnership working with healthcare professional and patient, while also promoting patient autonomy, as it is the person's goals (rather than the clinician's) that are the focus of care. For example, if one of Rosa's goals is to continue to be able to work for as long as possible, then interventions should be focused on enabling this to happen and addressing the barriers to this. Once goals are set, then steps can be taken towards the patient's goals. Goals should be reviewed when the patient's circumstances change.

Promotion of functioning

Earlier in the chapter we discussed how changes in functioning due to life-limiting illness will impact on people's ability to undertake their usual activities of daily living, with consequences for their health, wellbeing and quality of life. The goal or goals set by the patient should guide plans of care that promote the functioning required to achieve these goals. This will often involve input from different members of the interdisciplinary team. Working in this way may enhance communication and collaboration among the team, who have a shared focus for care and can promote effective use of services, with the patient being signposted to those services best able to address their needs (Fettes et al., 2018).

Promoting functioning requires nurses to consider an holistic, biopsychosocial perspective of health, and different members of the interprofessional team will have a role. Let's take Rosa as an example. Rosa has identified a short-term goal to have less pain in her hip so that she will be less irritable and can play with her children. Achieving this goal will involve a pain assessment to identify reasons for her hip pain and to address reversible causes. It may involve referral to physiotherapy and reviewing her use of analgesics, but also psychological support to explore her experiences of parenting while living with a life-limiting condition.

In the Useful websites section at the end of this chapter there is a link to a short film which demonstrates the rehabilitative approach to palliative care. Promoting functioning will often involve addressing troublesome symptoms, such as Rosa's hip pain.

Symptom management

Symptom management is considered synonymous to a palliative approach to care and is sometimes misunderstood by the public as the only focus of palliative care. Management of troublesome symptoms is very important, as these can significantly impact on quality of life and living well and cause distress for patients and their families. Finding out about symptoms, specifically which symptoms are distressing or problematic, will enable an appropriate plan of care to be developed to support the patient. Symptoms may be caused by the disease itself, be a side effect of treatments, or due to other causes such as comorbidity. Symptoms are often physically unpleasant, and the embodied experience of these will be further affected by the patient's interpretation of what the symptom 'means', as illustrated by Marc's experience from the time he received his cancer diagnosis, described below.

Case study: Marc

Marc had had a tickly cough on and off for years. As a younger man, he had worked in the mining industry and it was common that after a few shifts he and his mates would all joke about how they could feel the dust on their lungs. He was also a smoker until stopping in his 50s when his first grandchild was born. Despite giving up smoking, he would still get frequent chest infections that sometimes seemed to last all winter.

Marc's friend and neighbour had nagged him to visit the GP about his cough which she insisted had become worse than it used to be. Marc had also been losing a bit of weight and was more tired than normal, but he put that down to getting older.

His GP seemed more concerned about these things than he was, and strongly suggested that he get seen at the hospital, just to rule out anything serious. Everything seemed to move quickly from there on. Almost before he knew it a doctor was telling him that there was a tumour in his lung, and it was cancer.

Once he knew that he had cancer his cough felt different. Instead of just being part of who he was, it was now a painful sign that he is a cancer patient. Every time he coughed, he could feel people looking at him like he had a big label that said 'CANCER HERE'. He no longer felt like a 'proper' man, but someone ill and frail and anxious.

Marc's knowledge that the cough now indicated that he had cancer changed his experience of this. It made what had been a fairly regular and accepted part of his life into a symptom that was indicative of a serious life-threatening illness and made him feel exposed and vulnerable to what others thought of him. It had affected his self-identity and sense of dignity.

Problematic symptoms have a significant effect on wellbeing as they prevent people from living their usual, or preferred way of life. They can impact on the ability to undertake activities of daily living, of working (which may in turn affect financial security) and on relationships. Commonly experienced symptoms include pain, fatigue and nausea and vomiting, among others. In this textbook, we will not be exploring approaches to symptom management in depth and encourage you to read your local palliative care formularies and to explore the recommended reading for this chapter which offers detailed exploration of symptom management. Instead, we will give an overview of three of the most common symptoms here, considering why addressing symptoms is important to improve functioning and quality of life.

Pain

Pain is one of the most feared symptoms of illness and affects many people. This includes around three-quarters of people with cancer at some point in their illness (Watson et al., 2019). People with chronic diseases and dementia or frailty also experience pain. It is a commonly experienced symptom and one that can be particularly challenging to assess due to communication difficulties. Pain can often be under-assessed and under-treated in these groups of people (Lichtner et al., 2014).

Pain is a subjective experience; therefore, pain should be accepted as what the patient says it is to them. Many people will have more than one pain associated with an illness, and different pains can occur through the course of their illness. Rigorous and systematic assessment of pain is essential to try and identify the cause of the pain and to develop a plan in partnership with the patient to manage this.

Tools for practice: pain assessment

Pain assessment should occur frequently. On admission to a ward or service, a full pain assessment is required which may involve different members of the professional team. Regular reassessments should occur to evaluate the effectiveness of treatments – for example, when medication is administered as part of the ward round, or when community nurses visit to provide supportive care. Early identification and management of pain is important.

Pain assessment involves gathering information to understand the individual's experience of pain and how it is affecting them, its location, type (e.g., is it chronic, acute, persistent, fluctuating etc.?), what current treatments are (including prescribed medicines, non-prescribed medicines and any other interventions), whether they are effective and the patient's goals in relation to pain management.

Some people may benefit from having an advocate (often a family member) involved when you are doing the assessment. For example, people with learning disabilities or people with dementia may struggle to understand or communicate their experiences, so take time to explain what you are doing and consider whether families and carers should also be involved with the assessment.

Pain assessment involves gathering a range of information using questioning, listening, measurement and interpretation and observational skills (Ford, 2019). You need to speak to the person about the site(s) of their pain, when it occurs and what it feels like, how severe the pain is, whether anything helps to resolve or reduce pain. You should also seek to ascertain how the pain is impacting on their psychosocial health, wellbeing and quality of life. You should observe for non-verbal indicators of pain through the person's body language such as grimacing, wincing and changes to movement, and consider psychological factors such as low mood, irritability and social factors such as whether it is inhibiting them being involved in their usual activities and how it impacts on their relationships (Ford, 2019).

Most clinical areas will use pain assessment tools as part of this process. These include simple pain rating scales where '0' is no pain and '10' is the worst possible pain, and the patient is asked to give a number to their pain. You can see a pain rating scale in Figure 4.4.

Pain rating scales can be particularly useful to assess whether any interventions are being effective – for example, by obtaining a score when commencing any analgesia and then at review to see if the pain is worse, the same, improving or has resolved. Patient responses to rating scales need to be considered as part of the wider assessment of pain.

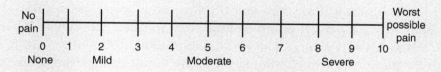

Figure 4.4 Example of a pain rating scale

Pain rating scales are an example of tools that support assessment of only one dimension of the pain (in this case, its severity). There are also multidimensional pain tools, which support assessment of the experience and implications of the pain, as well as measuring the severity and type of pain and identifying the area(s) in the body where it occurs.

Pain assessment is the first step in pain management. It needs to be followed by actions and interventions which will address pain.

Pain can usually be managed with commonly available non-opioid and opioid analgesics alongside non-pharmacological interventions. Unmanaged pain has many consequences and, when severe, can be very distressing to the patient, particularly when they think that this could be a sign that there is something seriously wrong with them. Acute and severe pain requires urgent intervention to identify the cause of the pain and to manage this as quickly as possible. Complex causes of pain, or pain that proves hard to manage, may require review from specialist teams to develop effective pain management strategies. Undertake Activity 4.5 to develop your understanding of pain assessment tools.

Activity 4.5   Exploring practice and simulation

Explore what pain assessment tools are used in your clinical placement area.

Simulate doing pain assessments with a student nurse colleague. Reflect on the benefits and limitations of the different tools, and the skills that you used to do the assessment.

There are no answers provided to this activity as it is based on your own practice.

The pain assessment tools you identified in Activity 4.5 may have included tools that explore different aspects of pain. Cicely Saunders, considered the founder of hospice care, famously introduced the concept of 'total pain'. Total pain includes physical pain, but also psychosocial, social, emotional and spiritual pain as well. Saunders suggested that to understand pain a clinician had to also understand the other elements of a patient's suffering and that truly listening to their story and their experience will help to identify their pain, and to work towards treating this.

The scenario involving Marc demonstrates the concept of 'total pain'. His cough caused him some discomfort, but his pain also linked to his changed self-identity, his sense of losing his masculinity and fear for a future in which he was frail. In order to help Marc with his pain, it would be important to listen carefully to his story and be a witness to his experience. The art of compassionate listening, and being present with a patient, can feel like doing very little, but it is immensely important for patient care.

Fatigue

Fatigue is the subjective experience of feeling persistently tired, weak and lacking energy that is not resolved by sleep or rest. Fatigue varies in severity and is highly prevalent in people with advanced disease. Despite this prevalence, the pathophysiology of fatigue remains poorly understood and there are limited pharmacological interventions with a weak evidence base for these (Mücke et al., 2015). There is some evidence that suggests physical exercise may be a beneficial intervention for people with cancer-related fatigue, but there is limited evidence for interventions for people with other diseases (Mochamat et al., 2021). This is a field in which there remains a need for better quality evidence. If people have persistent and enduring fatigue that is not responsive to primary care interventions, further assessment and support may be beneficial from specialist palliative care teams.

Nausea and vomiting

Nausea, the feeling of needing to vomit, and vomiting (or emesis) are common and can be caused by a wide range of factors including treatments (such as cytotoxic chemotherapies and opioids used for pain relief), metabolic disorders (like hypercalcemia or renal failure), gastric stasis, vestibular disturbance (a side effect from opioids or brain tumours) and anxiety (NICE, 2021a). Identifying the cause of nausea or vomiting enables an appropriate treatment plan to be developed. Nausea and vomiting may be short term, and often resolves with antiemetic (anti-sickness) medications and/or, where possible, addressing reversible causes. Persistent nausea or vomiting should be reassessed and, if not resolved within 24 hours, referral should be made to specialist palliative care teams for support (NICE, 2021a).

Identifying and managing problematic symptoms will help to improve functioning and reduce suffering and is an essential part of supporting people to have the best quality of life they can in their individual circumstances.

Chapter summary

This chapter has explored what it means to live well with a life-limiting, incurable illness and highlighted issues that are a threat to health and wellbeing. Typical trajectories of illness have been described including how a person's changing functional abilities may impact on their sense of dignity, wellbeing and quality of life. The activities in this chapter have encouraged you to reflect on the implications of living with illness and apply theory to case studies. The chapter has also introduced the rehabilitative model of palliative care which promotes individual autonomy, choice and independence through goal-setting and the promotion of functioning (including good symptom management) as a goal for care.

Activities: brief outline answers

Activity 4.4   Critical thinking (page 73)

Rosa has mentioned a few things that might be relevant to include in goal-setting conversations, including a wish to:

- live to see her children start school
- attend work
- undertake hobbies
- be a good mum
- reduce pain in the hip.

Further reading

Watson, M, Ward, S, Vallath, N, Wells, J and Campbell, R (2019) *Oxford Handbook of Palliative Care*. Oxford: Oxford University Press.

This handbook for nurses, doctors and others working in the field of palliative care contains comprehensive information about managing symptoms, and other core elements of palliative care practice.

Mitchell, W (2018) *Somebody I Used to Know*. London: Bloomsbury.

This *Sunday Times* bestseller explores the experiences of Wendy Mitchell who was diagnosed with dementia at the age of 58.

Useful websites

www.dyingwell.uk/

Clair Fisher had stage 4 bowel cancer. She developed this website to share her personal perspective of what it means to live well at the end of life.

You can also see Clair's twitter account @dyingwell_UK

https://youtu.be/eIEQOZEr3Lo

This short film explores the experience of Lucy who has COPD and receives a rehabilitative approach to her palliative care.

https://cks.nice.org.uk/specialities/palliative-care/

The National Institute for Clinical Excellence (NICE) has developed a range of palliative care *Clinical Knowledge Summaries* (CKS) which are regularly updated evidence-based guidance on addressing common symptoms.

Chapter 5 Complexity in palliative and end of life care

Chapter aims

After reading this chapter, you will be able to:

- understand what is meant by 'complexity'
- describe factors that contribute to complex support needs in palliative and end of life care

(Continued)

(Continued)

- explain the role of specialist palliative care in helping support people with complex care needs
- reflect on your personal strategies for self-care and discuss ways of developing and maintaining this.

Case study: Rachel

Rachel was spending the day with the specialist palliative care team who worked in the hospital. This morning they had been visiting the wards to support the staff there caring for people with complex support needs. This had included someone whose pain had been very difficult to resolve and someone who had both a learning disability and cervical cancer. In the afternoon, Rachel was going to attend an education session that the specialist nurse was delivering about palliative care to newly qualified nurses. Rachel was interested to see the role that the specialist nurse had, but also wondered whether specialist nurses were involved in the care of everyone who was at the end of life …

Introduction

When you first start working in healthcare, it can seem as though all the care that you are involved with is very complex. As you gain knowledge, develop your capabilities and experience throughout your education, you will start to recognise that all people who access healthcare have support needs, but that some of these are more difficult, or complex, to address than others.

In this chapter, we will explore what is meant by 'complex' needs and 'complexity' in palliative and end of life care. We will discuss the biopsychosocial-spiritual framework and use this as a tool to explore complex needs. You will then have opportunity to apply this to case studies as a framework to exploring the various support needs that people might have. We will explore **delirium** as a specific type of a complex need and consider, as examples, two groups of people who often have complex support needs: people who are homeless, and people who have a learning disability. Most support needs are met by generalist care services, but where support needs are more complex specialist palliative care services will also be involved, as observed by Rachel in the scenario above. We will discuss the role of specialist palliative care and explore Rachel's question about whether everyone sees specialist palliative care services.

Healthcare systems are also inherently complex, involving multiple different 'parts' (e.g., services, people and locations) which are connected and interact with each other. We will discuss the patient experience of this, consider why collaboration within and between services is required, and the significance of continuity of care for people who need palliative and end of life care.

Caring for people who are dying, and their families, can be very rewarding, but it involves emotional labour and can be personally challenging. To maintain personal wellbeing and standards of care nurses need to develop emotional intelligence and strategies for self-care and resilience; we will explore this at the end of this chapter.

Throughout this chapter we will use a range of mini scenarios to help to demonstrate the theory that we are discussing.

Complexity in care

Scenario: Mrs Zhang

We [the community nurses] are doing a risk assessment in relation to visiting Mrs Zhang, and are working with the GP, the community mental health team and social services to try and develop an appropriate care package to support her and work towards her goals. We have been told that Mrs Zhang speaks limited English and has complex needs. We know that she has a hoarding disorder and is known to mental health services. She also has advanced cancer and has expressed a preference to die at home. Her home is extremely full of things to such an extent that it is difficult to access the bathroom and kitchen, and there is only a small pathway to her bed.

There are many contributing factors to complexity in palliative and end of life care and some care needs and care situations are more complex to address than others. Before we start discussing complexity in care, do Activity 5.1 which encourages you to critically consider this concept.

Activity 5.1   Critical thinking

You may have read clinical referrals or heard healthcare practitioners referring to complex situations, or a person with complex care needs. You will also see this referred to in the NMC Standards of Proficiency. Spend a few minutes considering the following questions. What do you think 'complexity' is? What is 'complex care', or a 'complex situation' in palliative or end of life care? What are 'complex care' needs?

There are no answers provided to this activity as these are your own ideas. The following section will discuss these concepts and further your understanding of these issues.

Activity 5.1 encouraged you to consider what 'complexity' and 'complex' might mean in palliative and end of life care. There is no universal definition of a 'complex patient' or 'complexity' in healthcare (Pask et al., 2018; Manning and Gagnon, 2017) which can lead to this feeling like a difficult concept to understand. Over the next few pages, we will explore what 'complexity' and 'complex' mean and consider how thinking about complexity as a nurse can help you to adopt an holistic perspective on nursing practice.

In its simplest form, complexity means that there are lots of different 'parts' to something that interact with each other. In relation to someone's health, we can initially think of these parts as the different issues that contribute to biopsychosocial-spiritual health, and to the services a person interacts with. For example:

- **issues linked biological factors:** e.g., having an progressive life-limiting illness, multiple health problems (multimorbidity), a rare or difficult to treat illness, symptoms that are not well controlled, taking lots of different medications (polypharmacy). These factors may be new, or pre-existing;
- **issues linked to social factors:** e.g., the impact of the illness on a person's finances, poverty, their environment, employment and working conditions, relationships with family and friends, interactions with community networks, changes to personal, professional and familial roles, changing levels of independence with usual or self-care;
- **issues linked to psychological factors:** e.g., issues with adjusting to illness, coping, distress, changing sense of identity;
- **issues linked to spiritual factors:** e.g., issues related to meaning and purpose in life, religion, faith;
- **issues linked to service provision:** e.g., availability and accessibility of care providers, the number of services involved in care, waiting times for treatments, locations of services, competence of the workforce and other workforce pressures such as staff shortages.

These 'parts' or the different issues contributing to health are frequently linked. It is often the case that the greater the number of issues, or greater number of connections between the issues leads to increased complexity. Interventions that help to address one issue may have consequences for other issues in the person's life (both positive and negative) and in unpredictable ways.

Complexity can be seen in the scenario at the start of this section involving Mrs Zhang. She has multiple healthcare conditions (biological elements), a hoarding disorder (social and psychological elements), her home environment is difficult to safely provide nursing care within and there are multiple care providers involved (service provision). The level of complexity is exacerbated by the communication challenges, as Mrs Zhang relies on translators. The situation with Mrs Zhang will continue to develop, but we do not know what will happen next. It will depend on what interventions occur, how Mrs Zhang responds to these, how the services involved collaborate and how her health changes over time.

These dynamic interactions highlight the need for a palliative approach to care (Pask et al., 2018) which considers the whole-person experience.

We will now consider a different case which also explores the dynamic nature of complexity.

Case study: Grace

Grace is 80 and was admitted to hospital following a fall in her home on the stairs a fortnight ago. She has a medical history of moderate frailty, stage 3 heart failure and diabetes. Grace has been living on her own, with family support.

Grace was originally admitted to the ward for observation while she was started on antibiotics for a urine infection, but the initial stay has now been extended. Nurses on the ward have expressed surprise that Grace was living on her own as, although Grace sustained no serious injuries in the fall, Grace has been quite confused, sometimes doesn't remember where she is and has been trying to leave the ward. Her family have said that she is not normally like this; they are very worried about her. She has also been quite confrontational, particularly when the nurses have been monitoring her blood glucose, which she had refused to let them take today.

A student nurse, Erica, was working on the night shift and she noticed that Grace was very restless overnight and didn't appear to get much sleep. Grace got up at about 4 o'clock in the morning and sat in the chair next to her bed and would not be coaxed back to bed.

Erica offered Grace a cup of tea which was gratefully accepted, and Erica asked Grace if she could join her and they sat in the patient room with their drinks.

Grace started talking about how difficult she found it to sleep in the hospital and that she was exhausted. Grace had lived alone for the past ten years following the death of her husband and found the constant noises from the nurse's station, other patients talking at night or watching television on their computers or snoring, and the lights going on and off when people were admitted overnight to be making her anxious and she had not been getting much sleep at all. The ward routines were very different from her own – she didn't want a hot drink at 9.30 at night, or to lay in bed until 7am. She has always woken early as she spent her career working as a baker and had started work very early in the morning, but she also usually went to bed early in the evening, at around 8 o'clock. She was aware that during the day she was getting grumpy and sometimes would be very 'dozy'; she was also craving a cigarette. She was very worried that the nurses would think that she couldn't look after herself and would make her move into a nursing home. She had previously done advance care planning and been clear that she wanted to live at home until she died as this was where she felt closest to her husband. No-one on the ward had spoken to her about this. Grace felt like they were treating her like an old woman and as though she was stupid – they kept trying to do her blood glucose for her and even though she did get breathless sometimes, she was more than capable of doing this herself.

(Continued)

(Continued)

Erica spoke to her practice supervisor about the conversation. They asked Grace if she would prefer to be in a side room rather than the four-bedded bay that she was currently in, and whether she would like to start nicotine replacement therapy while she was in hospital, which Grace agreed to.

Over the next few days, the confusion resolved and Grace appeared to be like a different woman. Grace slept much better and the nurses agreed goals of care with Grace and discussed her wishes and preferences for future care. Grace was clear that she wanted to return home, so an occupational therapist visited Grace's house with her. They identified some risks in the house that may have contributed to her fall and, with help from her family, Grace was supported to move her bedroom downstairs so that she didn't have to go upstairs at night.

Grace was also referred to the community nurses, who agreed to visit Grace every few weeks to review how the new arrangements were working for Grace, and to support Grace to continue to achieve her goals.

Grace's case study involves a range of biopsychosocial-spiritual issues that are inter-related, affect each other and change over time. In Activity 5.2 you will apply the biopsychosocial-spiritual framework to Grace's situation and consider whether this is a complex care situation and why.

Activity 5.2 Application to practice

Re-read the case study involving Grace and then fill in the table below with the issues that are contributing to Grace's health during her hospital stay. You will probably need to continue this on an additional sheet of paper …

Biological issues	Psychological issues	Social issues	Spiritual issues	Service issues
e.g., stage 3 heart failure	*e.g., concern about being admitted to a nursing home*	*e.g., environment of the ward*	*e.g., desire to feel close to her husband by living at home*	*e.g., nurses taking blood glucose*

Once your table is complete, consider whether you think Grace's situation is complex and whether she has complex care needs?

Answers are provided at the end of the chapter.

In Activity 5.2 you will have identified that the complexity associated with Grace's situation changed throughout the course of her stay in hospital. There were issues that stretched across the biopsychosocial-spiritual domains which were further affected by the relationship with the nurses. As a result, there was interaction between the different 'parts' of Grace's situation – for example, the environment of the ward led to Grace not being able to sleep, feeling anxious and probably contributed to her being confused and disoriented.

In this section we have established that complexity occurs because people and healthcare services are complex; they contain multiple parts (across the biopsychosocial-spiritual domains and in service provision) that interact to create complex care situations that will evolve in unpredictable and dynamic ways. Proactive assessment and management of issues contributing to complexity, and consideration of how changes in one domain might impact on others, reduces the risks of negative outcomes. For example, if Grace's nurses had explored Grace's usual sleep routine as part of an holistic assessment on admission, and discussed her goals for care, then Grace's experience might have been different.

We have discussed a range of issues that contribute to complexity in care, and you have started to consider in Activity 5.2 whether Grace had complex support needs. We will now explore complex patient needs in greater detail.

Complex patient needs

A need arises where there is some aspect of a person's biopsychosocial-spiritual health where they have a problem or issue that they cannot address themselves and need support to do this. Needs arise out of the problems that people experience, and the goals that they want to achieve. For example, Grace had a fall which led to an acute hospital admission (a problem) and her overarching goal was to return home. Therefore, Grace had some support needs that related to how to safely achieve this goal, while also responding to her fluctuating support needs (arising out of additional problems and shorter-term goals) while in hospital.

A fundamental part of nursing practice is assessing a person's needs before planning, providing and evaluating care. People who are living with a progressive illness will experience changing support needs throughout their illness and at the end of life, and their goals will also change and develop alongside this. It is important to explore an individual's understanding of their needs rather than presuming that people have needs based on their diagnosis. This helps to ensure that care is person-centred.

While all patients have needs, complex needs are those which are more challenging to address. Pask et al. (2018) found that complexity was often cumulative – that is, problems experienced across multiple domains lead to increased complexity, but also recognised that complexity could sometimes be related to a single issue, such as uncontrolled pain, or being a single parent with dependents.

Complex needs are often seen in palliative care. Specialist palliative care, which we will discuss later in this chapter, has a significant role in supporting patients, families and services in relation to these.

There are many possible examples of complex support needs; in the following sections we have chosen three specific situations that you may encounter in practice. Delirium, palliative care for people who are homeless and palliative care for people who have a learning disability.

Complex patient needs: delirium

Delirium is an example of a single issue that is often complex as it has many possible causes, can be challenging to identify and to address and can be very distressing for patients and families. Delirium should be considered when someone presents with recent (over hours or days) unexplained changes in their behaviour, and an assessment undertaken by a professional with appropriate competence and training. Delirium is common in people who are receiving palliative care and becomes more common towards the end of life.

Delirium is categorised into three types: hyperactive, hypoactive and mixed (NICE, 2019). In hyperactive delirium, people may be restless, agitated, confused, have hallucinations, be paranoid, have sleep disturbance and experience changes to their usual communication or mood or personality. Hypoactive delirium is harder to recognise and may present as poorer concentration than usual, slow responses to questions, reduced mobility or movement, and social withdrawal. People with mixed delirium will have both hypoactive and hyperactive elements.

Causes of delirium may be complex and in palliative care contexts, include medications, drug withdrawal (including alcohol and nicotine), constipation, dehydration, urine retention, pain, sensory impairments, or liver or renal impairments, electrolyte disturbances, hypercalcaemia, infection, hypoxia and brain tumours among other factors (NHS Scotland, 2020).

Delirium is treated by identifying and addressing any reversible causes and by helping to orient the patient in their environment. It is important to provide reassurance as people with delirium may often be scared about what is happening. Effective communication can help to orient the patient, including about where they are, who you are and why they are here. A clock on the wall so people can see what time it is and avoiding moving people to other environments, if possible, can also help (NICE, 2019). Where causes of delirium are not reversible – for example, where someone is approaching the end of their life – local end of life care guidelines should be followed.

Complex patient needs: palliative care for people who are homeless

Case study: Mari

Mari is 40 and hasn't had a permanent home since a relationship breakdown six years ago. She has struggled with her mental health since young adulthood and is alcohol-dependent. Mari has advanced liver disease and the warden at the hostel has called an ambulance as she is in pain and is distressed.

People who are homeless and vulnerably housed experience complex health issues (like Mari, in the case above) which often include a mix of mental health, physical health and substance misuse and addiction-related problems. This is sometimes referred to as 'tri-morbidity' and contributes to the shocking statistic that people who are homeless have an average life expectancy that is 30 years shorter than the general population (Kennedy et al., 2018).

The complex needs of this group of people arise from their experiences. This includes those that may have led to them becoming homeless. These may include relationship breakdowns or the legacy of childhood abuse and trauma, their physical and mental health, substance misuse which is used as a coping strategy but contributes to physical health problems, and barriers to accessing healthcare which include stigma and discrimination (Lyons, 2021).

People who are part of the homeless community are also likely to have experienced the premature, unpredictable and sometimes unpleasant deaths of other community members, and this can shape their beliefs and understanding about dying and death. This may also lead to some people being fatalistic about death (accepting that it is just how it is) and others being very fearful of unpredictable or unpleasant deaths (James et al., 2021).

Usual palliative care services may struggle to meet the complex needs of people who have tri-morbidity, and this can lead to poor care experiences for people who are homeless which impacts their future help-seeking behaviours. Collaboration between services who routinely work with people who are homeless and generalist and specialist palliative care services is essential to improve appropriate access to palliative care. There is increasing work being done in this area and some hospices have developed collaborations with local homeless projects to raise awareness of what palliative care can offer, and to identify people who may benefit from palliative care support.

You can learn more about homelessness and palliative care by watching the film we have included in the recommended websites section at the end of this chapter.

Complex patient needs: palliative care for people with learning disabilities

People with learning disabilities also experience worse physical and mental health than the general population; on average someone with a learning disability's life expectancy is eighteen years shorter for women and fourteen years shorter for men than people who do not have a learning disability (NHS Digital, 2019). Reasons for this disparity are complicated, but include preventable deaths, lower rates of cancer screening, higher rates of some comorbidities such as severe mental illness and epilepsy and increased risk of developing some conditions, such as Alzheimer's disease in people who have Downs syndrome (NHS Digital, 2019).

Learning disabilities exist on a spectrum from mild to profound and people will have lived with their disability their whole life. In Activity 5.3 you will apply what you know about palliative and end of life care to considering the support needs of someone with a learning disability.

Activity 5.3   Application of knowledge to practice

Based on what you know about the challenges that people with learning disabilities experience and what you know about the end of life, what support needs do you think someone who has an advanced life-limiting illness and a learning disability might have? Why might these be complex?

There are no answers to this question as this is based on your own thoughts, but suggestions will be found in the following section.

People with a learning disability have complex needs due to their reduced ability to understand new or complex information, to learn new skills due to a reduced intellectual ability and to cope independently with everyday activities, such as household tasks and managing finances (Mencap, 2022). Marie Curie (2022b) highlights that people with a learning disability are more likely to:

- have unidentified health needs and complicated physical and mental health problems contributing to their requirements for palliative care;
- be diagnosed later than others leading to less time for palliative care intervention;
- find it difficult to understand information about their health and find transitions to new care settings difficult;
- struggle to communicate their needs, or how symptoms are affecting them, and to express their wishes and preferences for care.

The principles of palliative care remain the same whoever you are working with, and it is important that you see each person as an individual, whose expectations and concerns about the end of life will be shaped by their identity, culture, previous experiences and values and beliefs. When working with people who have a learning disability, it is especially important to involve families, friends and usual paid carers as partners in care, and to understand the person's communication preferences so that you can help people to understand their illness and what is happening to them, support them to communicate their experiences and explore what is important to them (NHS England, 2016). Creative approaches can be helpful in relieving distress and improving wellbeing (NHS England, 2017).

Box 5.1   Creative approaches to care: No Barriers Here

No Barriers Here is an innovative arts-based approach to advanced care planning which is used with people with learning disabilities and other people who experience unequal access to palliative care for reasons of identity, ethnicity, culture or race.

Learn more about this by exploring their page on twitter @NoBarriersHere and watching the film that is included in the recommended websites section at the end of the chapter.

The Palliative Care for People with Learning Disabilities Network has some excellent resources for developing your practice in this area. You will find the link to this in the Useful websites section of this chapter.

Our focus in this section has been on the person and their support needs. We will now go on to consider healthcare that exists to meet these needs, and some of the challenges of providing care in complex healthcare systems.

Healthcare provision and complex systems

Scenario: Tom

There are so many people coming to care for my partner, Tom, at home now that I am not sure who is in charge, or who to ring in an emergency.

Delivery of palliative care occurs within a complex healthcare system and there are numerous individuals, teams, services and organisations who have a stake in the care of people affected by life-limiting illness and at the end of life. Table 5.1 highlights some of these and you may be able to identify others as well.

Patients	Families	Lay-carers	Members of the patients' community
GPs	Specialist palliative care teams – community (nurses, doctors, AHPs)	Specialist palliative care teams – hospital (nurses, doctors, AHPs)	Hospice teams
Hospice at home teams	Marie Curie nurses and services	Macmillan nurses	Disease-specific specialist nurses
Ambulance services	Physiotherapists	Occupational therapists	Social workers
Social care providers (including home carers)	Chaplain and religious networks	Urgent and emergency care providers (e.g., A&E, out of hours doctors)	Bereavement services
Third sector organisations	The NHS	Private healthcare providers	The local authority

Table 5.1 Stakeholders affected by or involved with care delivery for people with advanced disease

While all these different individuals and organisations have a potentially important role to play in the delivery of palliative and end of life care, patients may find themselves involved with a bewildering array of different services. These are likely to be located in different places, with different (and sometimes unclear) roles in their care delivery and with different contact details and access arrangements. This is what Tom's wife was experiencing in the short scenario at the start of this section. Where care is not experienced as continuous or coordinated, there is a risk that patients and families experience this as fragmented and disjointed and may not know how to get help to address their needs. This lack of continuity also has implications for patient safety, increased use of urgent care services where people do not understand what service they should access, and care needs not being effectively met (den Herder-van der Eerden et al., 2017). Continuity of care, where patients experience their care as coherent, interconnected over time, consistent and aligned with their needs, wishes and preferences (WHO, 2018) is an aspiration of care organisations and is one of the intentions behind the development of **integrated care**.

The World Health Organization (2018) describes different types of continuity that will influence patients' and carers' experience of continuity across care settings.

- *Interpersonal continuity*, where continuous trusting relationships are developed among providers and receivers of care, and care is flexible and adapted to individual patient and family needs and that care is provided by the same central providers.
- *Longitudinal continuity*, where care is considered over time including discharge planning from admission, use of care navigators and clear referral strategies for healthcare professionals.
- *Management continuity*, where there is shared collaborative care by the interdisciplinary team, there is proactive and regular monitoring of long-term

conditions and that care planning considers the perspectives of multiple care providers (including crossing the boundaries of services and organisations).

- *Informational continuity*, where there is positive communication between patients and care providers, where healthcare records are shared and synchronised, that there are standardised clinical protocols across care settings and that information is shared among healthcare providers.

WHO (2018)

Activity 5.4 encourages you to apply the WHO (2018) perspective on continuity to your local healthcare context.

Activity 5.4   Exploring practice and critical thinking

Do some investigation into what services are available locally to support people with progressive illness and at the end of life. Remember to include NHS services, voluntary organisations and services in secondary and community settings (you might want to refer to Table 5.1 for ideas of whom to include). Make a list of these services.

Using the WHO (2018) different types of continuity, what challenges are there to providing continuity for patients and families locally?

Discuss with a student colleague any interventions or activities that you are aware of locally that aim to improve continuity for patients. An example of this might be community matrons or case managers to enable management continuity, or shared patient records to enable informational continuity.

There are no answers provided to this activity, as it is based on your own practice.

In Activity 5.4 you have considered what challenges there are locally to providing continuity of care. Collaboration between providers contributes to continuity.

Collaboration

Successful continuity of care between services relies on the people who work within these organisations collaborating (King et al., 2013). Collaboration requires effective communication, teamwork, having shared objectives and goals and respect for each other's role and profession (Emich, 2018). This may occur within professional groups, such as the nurses who work on a ward; in interdisciplinary teams, such as the specialist palliative care team; or in situations that cross organisational boundaries, such as collaboration between health and social care, or secondary care and primary care. In palliative care, collaboration will often also involve the patient, their carers and family in shared decision-making.

Nurses have an important role in supporting such collaboration.

Personalised care

Personalised care aims to give people more control over their own health and more personalised care when they need it (NHS, 2019) in order to deliver care that is sustainable, realistic and appropriate (QNI, 2022). This includes proactively identifying people who are in the last year of life so that care can be planned in partnership with them (NHS, 2019). Personalised approaches to care involve shared decision-making, personalised care and support planning, enabling choice, social prescribing, community-based support, supported self-management, personal health budgets and integrated personal budgets. This approach is particularly suited to people who are approaching the end of their lives after living with a long-term condition (including where cancer has been managed as a long-term condition) and is intended to reduce the challenges that complexity presents for people in these circumstances (NHS, 2019). Thinking of Grace's situation, she may have benefited from a personalised approach to her care. You can read more about NHS England's universal approach to personalised care on their webpages. We have included the link in the Useful websites section of this chapter.

Specialist palliative care

In palliative and end of life care many patient needs are met within general care services. These are healthcare services which do not specialise in palliative and end of life care but work with people affected by a range of problems. Examples of types of general care services include general practice, district and community nurses, pharmacies, general medical or surgical wards and urgent and acute services like A&E.

People whose needs or circumstances are more complex often benefit from specialist palliative care involvement and this should always be considered. We briefly introduced you to specialist palliative care in Chapter 1. Specialist palliative care is provided by care professionals whose sole focus of their work, and the service that they work in, is palliative and end of life care. These professionals will probably have received additional post-registration education and training to develop their skills and knowledge. Specialist palliative care provides services to patients, supports general care services to deliver care and provides education to the wider healthcare workforce.

Specialist palliative care services include hospices and the broad range of services that they provide, specialist nursing teams such as some Macmillan nurse and Marie Curie teams and specialist palliative care teams based in hospitals. Palliative medicine is a medical speciality whose doctors provide specialist palliative care.

Finucane et al. (2021) undertook a research study to explore the types of complex needs that were referred for specialist palliative care support. They found that most referrals had two or more 'needs' documented on the referral (with nearly half of referrals including six to ten needs, and 13 per cent including over eleven needs). Needs stated on referrals included pain, fatigue, shortness of breath, complex pain, agitation, confusion, fluctuating dynamic need, family or carer support, functional care needs, future planning, patient or family preference for referral and capacity or communication needs. This study demonstrates the cumulative nature of complexity (as most referrals included multiple support needs) which was also found by Carduff et al. (2018), who highlight that it is not only the number of needs that people have, but also how these different needs interact with each other. Examples of this include where psychological, social or spiritual needs interact with physical needs that lead to those needs becoming complex and requiring specialist intervention and support.

Specialist palliative care is generally provided through three main mechanisms in the UK (NHS England, 2016). The first is in liaison with the patient's usual care team (be that their care team in the hospital, or community); in these circumstances the clinical responsibility for care remains with the person's consultant or GP. In this type of involvement, a specialist assessment could be undertaken, the patient may be discussed at palliative care multidisciplinary meetings and recommendations given directly to the patient or to the usual care team. The second mechanism is through specialist in-patient palliative care. This may occur in a palliative care unit in hospitals or a hospice and sometimes in other settings. All care to the person is provided by people who specialise in palliative care. The third mechanism is specialist out-patient services where people have their needs assessed and care planned by specialists working in out-patient clinics or day centres. Care might be delivered by a range of professionals from the interdisciplinary team including medical, nursing, allied health professionals and social work. In these scenarios accountability for care is shared between the specialist clinicians and the primary care team.

As a nurse, you will encounter other challenges in providing good palliative care. These include developing your own skills and knowledge, the workforce pressures you encounter in practice and maintaining your own wellbeing.

Nursing: capability and the importance of self-care

Case study: Fynn

Fynn had been working the night shift on the medical ward. It had been very busy, with several admissions and with two people who were likely to be in the last days of life. They had been short staffed due to nursing vacancies, on top of which a nurse had called in sick. An extra nurse had been drafted in to join the shift but had said they did not feel confident providing end of life care as they usually worked in the out-patient's department. Fynn felt extremely tired and frustrated that he had not had the time he wanted to spend with the patients and their families. He was not sure how long he could keep doing this for.

Cases like the one involving Fynn above can be very challenging for nurses. Both Fynn, and the agency nurse, may have felt that they were unable to practise in line with their values due to the situation they were in. We will explore two issues highlighted by this scenario:

1. the capability of nurses to provide care; and

2. the importance of self-care.

Capability

If a nurse is capable, this suggests that they are they competent – thus having the knowledge, skills and attitude to practise safely – and that they also can adapt to change and continue to improve their performance (Fraser and Greenhalgh, 2001; Hanks et al., 2021). Being able to adapt to change, and apply knowledge and skills to evolving, or new scenarios are important attributes for successful and safe nursing practice for people with complex needs.

Where nurses (and other healthcare professionals) lack confidence and/or competence in palliative care they may perceive patient needs to be particularly complex (Carduff et al., 2018).

Developing your capability

Nursing involves lifelong learning and a commitment to personal development. As part of revalidation, nurses are required to undertake a minimum of 35 hours of continuing professional development, of which at least twenty hours must include participatory learning (NMC, 2021). There are many ways to develop your capability in providing palliative care throughout your career.

As a student, reading textbooks and engaging in the learning activities within them (such as those in this book!) and actively participating in learning opportunities at your university are good ways to develop your knowledge. While on placement, explore whether it is possible to spend time working with people who are living with life-limiting illness or at the end of life. It may also be possible to negotiate with your practice assessor to visit other services who provide specialist palliative care or spend time shadowing specialist palliative care nurses or other members of the multidisciplinary team.

Once you have graduated and registered as a nurse you will be able to access different types of learning opportunities. This might include training provided by your local palliative care team or hospice and post-registration courses offered through your local university (costs of which will vary depending on local agreements) which might include short courses, Master's degrees or PhDs. There are also now an increasing number of free online learning opportunities. For example, eLearning for health offers an End of Life Care for All programme and FutureLearn, in partnership with the University of Glasgow, offers End of Life Care: Challenges and Innovation. We have included links to these in the Useful websites section at the end of this chapter.

Training and education are important to develop your capability. Having a sustained and enjoyable career will also involve you developing robust strategies for self-care.

Self-care

Nursing people who live with advanced life-limiting illnesses and those at the end of life involves physically and emotionally demanding work in sometimes stressful and unpredictable situations. Developing strategies to care for yourself and to maintain your own wellbeing will support you to cope with the demands of the role. Everyone will find different techniques useful for self-care and Activity 5.5 encourages you to do some more reading around self-care and nurse wellbeing, before reflecting on your current self-care and considering future strategies for self-care.

Activity 5.5 Reading and reflection

Read the following article which is published in the *Nursing Times*. You should be able to access this through your university:

Cedar, D and Walker, G (2020) Protecting the wellbeing of nurses providing end-of-life care. *Nursing Times*, 116(2): 36–40.

Once you have read the article, reflect on your current strategies for self-care and consider what else you might do in your personal or professional life that will help to maintain your wellbeing.

When you did Activity 5.5, you may have found that you already have a strong strategy for self-care, or that you need to develop this further. It can feel difficult to prioritise caring for yourself when there are many demands on your time, but it is important to do so to maintain your own health. It is hard to provide good care for others, when you don't provide good care for you! Healthcare and higher education organisations increasingly recognise the importance of promoting the wellbeing of their staff. Activity 5.6 encourages you to explore what is available to you in the organisations you work within.

Activity 5.6 Exploring practice

Find out what the organisation that is hosting your placement offers in terms of wellbeing initiatives. You might find this information from staff notice boards, or webpages, or from speaking with your practice assessors, supervisors and other colleagues. Explore whether you can be involved with any activities and consider whether they may enhance your existing self-care strategies.

(Continued)

(Continued)

Repeat this activity but exploring what your university offers to support students with their wellbeing.

There are no answers provided for this activity as it is based on your own investigation.

Activity 5.6 highlights that, as a student nurse, you have links with different organisations which will include your university and the healthcare organisations that you have placements with. Accessing support to develop your self-care strategies and your wellbeing is good practice for your future career. Self-care is a vital part of your nursing practice which will help you to care for people with **emotional intelligence** (Heffernan et al., 2010), compassion and **resilience**.

Chapter summary

People have complex support needs because of the different aspects of their biopsychosocial-spiritual health which interact and affect each other. Most support needs are met within general healthcare services, but where needs become more complex specialist palliative care providers should be involved. Complexity also exists in healthcare because of the many different 'parts' of healthcare systems that interact with each other. Collaboration between care providers is required to provide continuity of care for patients who may need support to navigate the multiple services that are involved in their care.

Nursing within a complex healthcare system and supporting people who live with life-limiting illnesses or at the end of life is physically and emotionally demanding. It is essential that nurses develop strategies for self-care to maintain their own wellbeing and to enable them to provide quality care.

Activities: brief outline answers

Activity 5.2   Application to practice (page 86)

A range of issues are present in the case study involving Grace. We have included a list below, but this is not exhaustive and you may have included other issues as well.

Grace does have complex support needs as she has a range of issues across the biopsychosocial-spiritual spheres. Grace is experiencing cumulative complexity, whereby the number of issues to address has added to the complexity of her situation. The level of complexity in Grace's situation changes over the course of the scenario and becomes less challenging to address.

Biological issues:

- stage 3 heart failure
- diabetes
- multimorbidity

- probable polypharmacy
- urine infection
- on antibiotics
- confusion
- nicotine dependency
- 80 years old
- not sleeping well in hospital: lack of sleep contributing to confusion during the day
- possible delirium.

Psychological issues:

- frustrated with nursing staff
- fear of losing her autonomy and being forced to move out of her home
- not sleeping well in hospital: environmental noise causing her anxiety.

Social issues:

- usually lives alone and sleeps upstairs
- bereaved
- usually self-manages diabetes
- has family support
- not sleeping well in hospital: not used to being near other people sleeping
- regularly smokes.

Spiritual issues:

- wishes to be at home as she feels near to her husband there.

Service issues:

- relationship with the nurses
- availability of occupational therapist and community nurses
- has previously undertaken advance care planning, but it is unclear who this is shared with, or what other services are involved with Grace's care.

Further reading

WHO (2018) *Continuity and Coordination of Care: A Practice Brief to Support Implementation of the WHO Framework on Integrated People-centred Health Services*. Available online at: apps.who.int/iris/bitstream/handle/10665/274628/9789241514033-eng.pdf (accessed 21 October 2022).

This practice brief explores continuity and coordination of care and gives global examples of interventions aimed to improve these aspects of care.

Useful websites

www.england.nhs.uk/personalisedcare/comprehensive-model/

These webpages provide an overview of NHS England's vision of universal personalised care.

youtu.be/SZEfBkI7mao

Homlessness and Palliative Care. This excellent film explores issues of homelessness and palliative care.

youtu.be/G-ToRCT3UiU

No Barriers Here. This short film explores the arts-based No Barriers Here approach to advance care planning.

www.pcpld.org/

The Palliative Care for People with Learning Disabilities Network has useful information and resources to help develop your knowledge.

www.e-lfh.org.uk/programmes/end-of-life-care/

Free to access eLearning for health programme on End of Life Care for All.

www.futurelearn.com/courses/end-of-life-care

Free to access Future Learn programme End of Life Care: Challenges and Innovation.

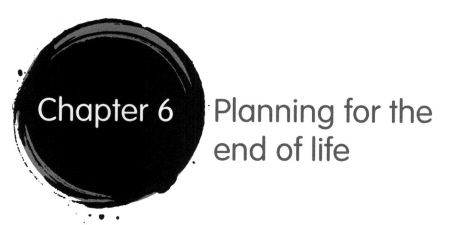

Chapter 6 Planning for the end of life

Chapter aims

After reading this chapter, you will:

- have understanding about why and how people might plan for their end of life
- have explored the debates about when planning for the end of life should occur
- have knowledge of what advance care planning is
- be aware of the different elements of end of life care planning including advance decisions to refuse treatment (ADRT), do not attempt cardiopulmonary resuscitation (DNACPR) orders and lasting power of attorney (LPA)
- have considered whose role it is to initiate advance care planning conversations.

Case study: Kai

Kai is in the final year of her undergraduate nursing degree. She has enjoyed her course and has experienced interesting and varied clinical placements. Kai has been involved in the care of a number of people who have been at the end of life during the past three years, but never very closely. A few months ago Kai's uncle Lei was diagnosed with motor neurone disease (MND) which is progressing rapidly. As the nurse in the family, she is being asked by her uncle about how he might start to plan for the things he knows are likely to happen to him as his illness progresses. Kai has heard people talking about planning for the palliative phase of an illness, but doesn't know too much about it. She promises her uncle that she will find out more.

Introduction

We spend much of our life planning. We make lists, we plan holidays, arrange gatherings for birthday celebrations, agree to meet friends and celebrate religious festivals. We think about our careers and the route we might like them to take. We may often have conversations with others in which we discuss our own plans for life and of theirs too. In general, more or less, we are quite good at planning! One of the things we are generally less good at is thinking and talking about the end of our lives; we are often too busy with living to think about what might be important to us when we are dying.

Given that we will all die, it is interesting to reflect how little time we may spend thinking and planning for it. One of the fundamental things that we can do is make a will outlining what might happen to property, money and other assets after we die. However, it is estimated that only 41 per cent of adults in the UK have written a will, which is perhaps representative of a broader lack planning for the end of life (Wealth Adviser, 2020).

Some may think it is morbid to think about death, or too sad to think about how life might be without either themselves or someone they love as part of it. However, as Kathryn Mannix eloquently describes, *Talking about death won't make it happen, but not talking about it robs us of choices and moments that will not come again* (Mannix, 2021, p. 142).

This chapter aims to provide you with information about the formal mechanisms involved with planning for what might happen at the end of life, including discussions about cardiopulmonary resuscitation (CPR), treatment escalation plans (TEPs), advance decisions to refuse treatment (ADRTs) and advance care planning (ACP). We will also explore some of the ways in which you can be involved with supporting people to think about their future wishes and preferences through careful listening. This involves being open and curious to the views and experiences of the patients you work with and care for. We will also briefly discuss assisted suicide and euthanasia, highlighting the developing debates in this area and how these may link to planning for future conversations.

Planning ahead

Increasingly, we are starting to see a greater public awareness about thinking about 'what matters' in life, including in illness and as someone approaches the end of life. This has been promoted through public health campaign such as the 'What matters to you' annual day in June and the End of Life Think Tank's (2021) online resources, which we have included in the recommended websites section of this chapter. Recent interest may be in part due to the Covid-19 pandemic that started in March 2020, when people were confronted with significant uncertainties about infection, hospitalisation, severe illness and the untimely and unexpected death of many tens of thousands of people.

What has begun to emerge from this are gentle suggestions about considering what matters to you and those you love, both in everyday life and if confronted with ill health and possibly the end of life. Asking the question, 'What matters to me?' both of ourselves and those around us, supports our planning for the future and can help us to feel more in control of our choices.

The following activity invites you to reflect on what matters to you in life, and whether people close to you may know this?

Activity 6.1   Reflection

Think about what matters most to you in your life right now. It might be family, friends, your pets, your university course, your hobbies, places you visit etc. …

When you have thought about these things, next consider how much those close to you know about what matters to you.

(Continued)

(Continued)

Make some notes of your answers.

We have not provided answers to these questions as they are your own thoughts on these issues.

Thinking about what matters to you is really important. Hopefully, you are doing this from a position of having relatively good health and wellbeing. If that changed, however, or you are facing ill health or living with a long-term condition, it is worth thinking about how you think what matters to you might change, or how it did alter if you've previously experienced a change in your own health.

How people's thoughts may change over time presents some of the challenges that are associated with planning ahead. To have things too firmly established can lead to disappointments or frustrations if situations and circumstances change that mean that our plans don't come to fruition. When we place planning ahead in the context of ill health, this adds a further layer of complexity. When people receive a diagnosis that means their life is now limited in terms of time, or they become seriously ill, what matters to them often changes; priorities get reordered and redefined, and things that seemed very important before can start to feel much less significant. What they had planned for before may all now change. We discussed the planning of care in Chapter 4 – specifically looking at person-centred goal-setting, where patients and healthcare professionals work together to establish what matters to the patient and what they hope to achieve in their life, and use this to plan current interventions that help the patient progress towards these goals. In this chapter we will explore advance care planning, where, from their current perspective, an individual thinks about what their preferences might be for their future care and at the end of life.

In thinking about planning for future care there are a number of formal processes and documents which you may come across in your clinical practice. It is helpful for you to have an understanding of these and what each of them signifies. We will outline these below, and will then start to think about how you, as a nurse, might find out if someone has such documents in place, alongside supporting someone to talk about their future plans.

Do not attempt cardiopulmonary resuscitation (DNACPR)

Cardiopulmonary resuscitation (CPR) is an intervention which attempts to restart someone's heart when they have experienced a cardiac arrest. CPR is an invasive intervention which involves chest compressions, delivery of high-voltage electric shocks across the chest, ventilation of the lungs and the intravenous injection of drugs.

For some individuals CPR is a successful intervention, but the likelihood of success varies greatly according to individual circumstances. Many of the processes involved in a CPR attempt are invasive and when successful can leave people with serious or long-term after-effects. CPR restarts the heart and/or breathing for between one and two in ten people whose heart or breathing have stopped. Overall, in England if you have a cardiac arrest out of hospital and emergency medical services undertake resuscitation, there is 7–8 per cent average survival to subsequent hospital discharge (NICE, 2018). Around a quarter of people in hospital who are treated by the hospital resuscitation team will survive until hospital discharge (Perkins et al., 2021). People can continue to be unwell after this and experience health consequences of the resuscitation, including neurological difficulties. People with existing complex health issues (such as those with advanced life-limiting illness) are much less likely to achieve a positive outcome of CPR.

As a result of this it is important to consider whether, in the event that someone's heart or breathing stops, they would like CPR to be conducted. For someone living with a life-limiting illness, the adverse effects of CPR and the limited likelihood of success may mean that they would not want CPR attempted on them. This will, however, be an individual decision.

It is a legal requirement for healthcare professionals who are considering making a DNACPR recommendation for an individual to discuss this consideration with that individual. It may be necessary for that discussion to happen with someone close to the patient as they themselves aren't able to be involved in that discussion due to an altered state of consciousness or they lack mental capacity (see the section on powers of attorney below). There is guidance available from the British Medical Association, the Resuscitation Council (UK) and the Royal College of Nursing (Resuscitation Council, 2016) which emphasises the absolute importance of these conversations occurring in order that decisions are made in the most informed way possible. The decision is then usually recorded in a form, which is shared with other healthcare professionals.

It is important to remember that healthcare professionals can make a DNACPR decision on behalf of a patient where a clinical decision has been made that CPR should not be attempted because it will not be successful (Resuscitation Council, 2016). However, it is required that the decision is clearly communicated and discussed with the patient and/or their family. So, while explicit consent for DNACPR is not required, what is vital is that there is consultation and communication wherever possible with the patient and their family.

It is also important to remember that if someone has a DNACPR decision, they should still be offered all other treatments that are appropriate in relation to their illness, including other types of life-sustaining treatment, and treatment to keep them pain-free and comfortable. An individual can also change their mind about having a DNACPR instruction in place.

Some people choose to have a DNACPR in place because they do not want to be resuscitated in an emergency, no matter what their health status. Others may make the decision to have a DNACPR in response to a change in their health, a new diagnosis, or a deterioration in a long-term condition. A DNACPR is possibly one of the more frequently encountered documents around end of life planning.

> ### Concept summary: responsibility for CPR and DNACPR decision-making
>
> *The overall clinical responsibility for decisions about CPR, including DNACPR decisions, rests with the most senior clinician responsible for the person's care as defined explicitly by local policy. This could be a consultant, general practitioner (GP) or suitably experienced and competent nurse. He or she should always be prepared to discuss a CPR decision with other healthcare professionals involved in the person's care. Wherever possible and appropriate, a decision about CPR should be agreed with the whole healthcare team.*
>
> Resuscitation Council (2016, p. 26)

Where a DNACPR decision gets recorded varies between settings. In some health and social care settings, DNACPR recommendations are recorded on a form that is specific only to a decision about DNACPR. However, many organisations and communities have moved to the use of broader emergency care plans such as treatment escalation plans.

Treatment escalation plans

A treatment escalation plan (TEP) is a document that details the treatments an individual may or may not want in the event that they become increasingly unwell and their condition deteriorates. They are particularly important for someone with advanced illness or nearing the end of their life, when treatment or escalation to intensive care may be seen as unlikely to have a positive outcome for the individual's health, or is contrary to a person's wishes. As with all forms of advance planning, TEPs should be thought through and discussed with a patient and their family and should be individualised, based on realistic goals of care for them.

An increasingly used example of a TEP is the Resuscitation Council UK Recommended Summary Plan for Emergency Care and Treatment (ReSPECT). It is used in a number of locations across the UK – although, at the time of writing, by no means all. The aim of using the ReSPECT documentation is to create an individualised plan of care and treatment in the case of an emergency situation where a person is unable to make or express their own care choices. The ReSPECT process can be used by anyone wishing to record their care wishes; however, like all TEPs, it may be most relevant to people who have complex health needs, are nearing the end of their lives, or who are at risk of sudden deterioration or cardiac arrest. This documentation can be particularly useful for paramedics if they are called out to a person who is receiving palliative care and helps to ensure that a patient's wishes are communicated.

A ReSPECT document should be completed as part of conversations between an individual, their families and the health and care professionals who are looking after them to understand what matters in terms of future care and treatment for that individual. As a result of these discussions, an individual's preferences and clinical recommendations are recorded on the non-legally binding form. It is important to remember that these decisions can and should be reviewed and adapted if an individual's circumstances change. We have included a link to the ReSPECT document in the Useful websites section of this chapter.

TEPs also present an opportunity to record whether the person has appointed a power of attorney.

Power of attorney

Power of attorney is the legal authority to make decisions on another person's behalf, either temporarily, or if someone loses mental capacity. Without power of attorney, it is not possible for someone to act on another person's behalf no matter what their relationship is to them. While there are slightly different laws around power of attorney across the four nations of the UK, the principles of power of attorney are similar in as much as they enable a process of formal representation of another person.

There are differing forms of power of attorney – for the most up to date information for each of the four UK nations, please do visit the relevant government power of attorney websites listed at the end of the chapter.

An **ordinary power of attorney (OPA)** allows one or more persons to make financial decisions on someone else's behalf. An OPA is only valid while an individual has the mental capacity to make their own decisions. It is suitable for someone who temporarily needs someone to act on their behalf – for example, if they are admitted to hospital, or if they are unable to access the bank or post office to manage financial affairs.

A **lasting power of attorney (LPA)** is a way of giving an individual the legal authority to make decisions on someone else's behalf should that person lose the mental capacity to make their own decisions at some point in the future, or if they no longer wish to make decisions for themselves. An LPA may cover both financial and health and social care decision-making.

As a student nurse it is important for you to know if someone has a lasting power of attorney in place and, if they do, what aspects of decision-making are contained within that. It is important also to establish whether or not a person has the capacity to make their own decisions, prior to any attorney they have appointed being asked to do so.

Enduring power of attorney (EPA) was replaced by LPA in October 2007; however, those made before that date are still valid and cover decision-making around property and financial affairs.

Concept summary: mental capacity and the Mental Capacity Act (NHS, 2021)

Mental capacity means having the ability to make or communicate specific decisions at the point at which they need to be made. To have mental capacity an individual must be able to understand the decision they need to make, why it needs to be made and the likely outcome of their decision.

The Mental Capacity Act (MCA) is designed to protect and empower people who may lack the mental capacity to make their own decisions about their care and treatment. It applies to people aged sixteen and over.

It covers decisions about day-to-day things like what to wear or what to buy for the weekly shop, or serious life-changing decisions like whether to move into a care home or have major surgery. Someone can lack capacity to make some decisions (for example, to decide on complex financial issues), but still have the capacity to make other decisions (for example, to decide what items to buy at the weekly shop).

The Mental Capacity Act (2005) says:

- Assume a person has the capacity to make a decision themselves, unless it's proved otherwise.
- Wherever possible, help people to make their own decisions.
- Do not treat a person as lacking the capacity to make a decision just because they make an unwise decision.
- If you make a decision for someone who does not have capacity, it must be in their best interests.

Treatment and care provided to someone who lacks capacity should be the least restrictive of their basic rights and freedoms. The NHS webpages provide accessible information about these issues. You can find a link to these webpages in the Useful websites section of this chapter.

Advance decision to refuse treatment (ADRT)

An advance decision to refuse treatment (ADRT), sometimes also known as an advance directive or living will, is a form of decision that can be made to refuse a specific type of treatment at some time in the future.

It lets an individual's family, carers and health professionals know about an individual's wishes to refuse specific treatments in the event that person becomes unable to make or communicate decisions by themselves.

Any treatments or interventions an individual wishes to refuse must be named in the advance decision. This can require some considerable thought. It is important for any decision to be discussed in detail with a healthcare professional in order that the full consequences of refusing a treatment are known. For example, an individual may say they wish to refuse all antibiotic treatment in the future. However, on further consideration they may wish to have antibiotics to treat a urine infection, which may cause severe discomfort, but not be life threatening, but choose to refuse antibiotics to treat a chest infection, which may be. Any refusal of life-sustaining treatments in circumstances where someone might die as a result needs to include a statement within the document that the advance decision applies even if it puts the individual's life at risk. Any individual can make an advance decision, as long as they have the mental capacity to do so.

In order for a decision to refuse life-sustaining treatment in the future to be legally binding the advance decision needs to be: written down, signed by the individual it relates to and signed by a witness. People who have made an ADRT should share this with their healthcare team. Many charities supporting people with life-limiting illnesses provide user friendly information for the public about ADRTs, and some, such as the Alzheimer's Society, provide templates to support people to record advance decisions to refuse treatment (Alzheimer's Society, 2021).

Advance care planning

Advance care planning (ACP) is a form of planning for future healthcare and treatment, which, while it can include many of the areas of advance planning discussed in the sections above, is broader in its scope. In its original form, ACP mainly involved the development of ADRTs enabling people to state if there were particular treatments or interventions they wouldn't want to receive in the future (Rietjens et al., 2021). Since its early beginnings, ACP has evolved into a process which includes much broader discussions that ideally take place over time and are revisited and revised (Hopkins et al., 2020).

Alongside the focus on future treatment wishes, ACP discussions can also include aspects of where someone might wish to live if they are unable to continue living at home, where they may wish to be cared for if they become unwell, often referred to as a 'preferred place of care'. They can also include considerations of where someone may wish to be cared for at the very end of their life (their preferred place of death) and it is important to bear in mind that this may be different to their preferred place of care (Sathiananthan et al., 2021). Ensuring that someone is enabled to die in the place of their choosing is one of the key quality indicators of the NHS Long Term Plan for England (NHS, 2019, p. 25), but perhaps more importantly it ensures that an individual has choice and control over their own death which may be important for their sense of dignity and their wellbeing.

Completing ACP documentation helps to ensure that family, healthcare professionals and others close to an individual are aware of an individual's wishes. Having these conversations early in the course of an illness can avoid situations occurring where decisions need to be made quickly and when it may be too late to ensure that what matters to someone can actually happen. Having an ACP can also help to avoid people being transferred into hospital for treatment they may not want and potentially dying there, rather than remaining at home or being transferred to a hospice.

Concept summary: advance care planning

ACP is a process that has been adopted internationally and, as such, has had a definition developed to ensure that there is consensus in understanding:

> *ACP enables individuals to define goals and preferences for future medical treatment and care, to discuss these goals and preferences with family and healthcare providers, and to record and review these preferences if appropriate.*
>
> Rietjens et al. (2017, p. e546)

Making our wishes known while we are well with regard to what matters to us in the future, or after receiving the diagnosis of an illness seems to make a lot of sense. In making plans, the people around us whom we care about will know what we want, won't have to guess on our behalf and, by thinking ahead, we can perhaps have some control over what then unfolds. We know, however, that people find talking about future plans around ill health and the end of life difficult. When someone is unwell, there are understandably some barriers that can prevent them from thinking about planning ahead. Reitjens et al. (2021) looked at the literature discussing some of the challenges that patients and healthcare professionals face in having advance planning conversations; we have outlined these challenges below.

Patients

- They may not be aware or may be uncertain about how ill they actually are.
- Their disease may have an unpredictable course and so it is difficult for them to determine when might be the right time to have such a conversation (we talked of different illness trajectories in Chapter 4).
- Equally, a person can know how unwell they are, but really not wish to believe this (i.e., be in denial) or may just not wish to talk about it.
- They may be waiting for the doctor or nurse to start a conversation about future healthcare plans with them, thinking that it is their job to do so.

Healthcare professionals

- They, too, may worry about the right time in a person's illness to raise the issue of advance planning. This may be for fear of raising something that hasn't previously been considered, of causing a person distress, or of causing them to lose hope.

- Finding the right time or enough time to have a conversation that needs to be well paced and considered may also be a concern.
- They may not feel well trained or prepared enough to have such conversations.

Rietjens et al. (2021)

These are all important considerations; however, we have not included these to put you off and make having a conversation about advance care planning seem too daunting. We highlight these points to make you aware of some of the concerns you and the people you care for may have about having such conversations. What is important for you to consider is how you, as a student nurse and future registrant, can help support people to think about advance care planning and to pick up cues that might tell you they are ready to talk about their future plans. There are practical aspects to consider also, including how advance care planning is documented in the clinical areas in which you work. Activity 6.2 asks you to begin to explore how advance care planning is documented in your clinical placement areas to start to develop your understanding of this.

Activity 6.2 Exploring practice and decision-making

When you are next on your clinical placement, find out what documentation is used in that health or social care setting to support people's decision-making around advance care planning and how these decisions are recorded. These documents may include those for DNACPR, ADRT and advance care planning.

We have not provided an answer to this activity as it will be individual to your clinical placement areas.

In Activity 6.2 you will have identified documentation relevant to your local organisations. It is important to remember when exploring the types of documentation used in health and social care settings that record people's future care wishes, that the documentation has been created as a result of conversations about future care plans. The following section discusses the importance of these conversations.

Conversations about future plans and the importance of listening

As we mentioned earlier, having conversations about future plans for care should ideally take place over a period of time and be discussions that are revisited with a trusted health professional. This may be an individual's GP or practice nurse, a community or specialist nurse visiting the patient at home. They may also be conversations that get started when someone is in hospital following admission with an unexpected illness or deterioration of a long-term, or life-limiting condition. In these circumstances the individual may be less well known to the nursing or other healthcare staff and conversations may need to be conducted over a shorter time frame. As a student nurse you may be present for part or all of these conversations. Equally, you may be caring for someone as they start to talk about the future course their illness might take and the uncertainties that might bring for them.

You will be taught communication skills as part of your nursing course; let's take a moment to think about what can help this type of conversation go well.

Activity 6.3   Reflective practice and communication

Think back to a conversation you have observed in clinical practice that covered a difficult to approach subject matter – for example, the delivery of a diagnosis or a test result to a patient or their relative.

Make a list of the factors that may have contributed to the conversation going well, and any that may have made it more challenging. Think broadly about this – the factors may include the physical location of where the conversation took place, the time available etc., in addition to the words used.

There is no answer provided for this activity as it is based on your own experience.

It is helpful to use the reflections identified in Activity 6.3 in thinking about how you can help support people in talking to you about their future plans. This may be a conversation about the possible trajectory their illness might take and thoughts they may have about their future care given this trajectory. In the section below we explore how you may support both the patient and yourself through such conversations.

In Chapter 4 we discussed different typical trajectories of illness and you may want to revisit that chapter to place the discussions here in the context of the courses that different illnesses can take.

Some patients may be very open about having a discussion about their future illness with you, feel confident about having that conversation and invite you into it. Where this happens, try and feel confident about engaging with them in return. Most likely it will require you to listen with understanding and remain curious through the conversation.

Kathryn Mannix (2021) talks in her book *Listen* about the idea of *listening with understanding*. Listening with understanding means the person who wants to talk to you and to whom you are listening feels that what they are saying to you is both important and understood.

You can do this by, first, letting the person know that you have time to listen to them, often by positioning yourself in a way that encourages someone to talk and, if appropriate, taking the time to pull up a chair. This simple action demonstrates that you have time to spend with them, helps you to share eye contact and changes the dynamics of a conversation by putting you both at a similar level. You may perhaps need to pause what you are doing if it is a task that takes you away from listening, like checking their observations. Or you may want to continue a task that facilitates listening-by-doing, such as supporting someone to have a wash. Give the person a cue that you are ready for them to continue, using phrases such as 'I'm happy to listen' or 'Where would like to start?'

If you do not have time to have a discussion when a patient indicates that they wish to talk, ensure that you communicate to the patient that you will make time and tell them when this will be and stick to it. For example: 'I am really happy to have a discussion with you and listen to your concerns; however, I am busy for the next hour. I will come back in an hour and we can talk then. Is that OK with you?'

As the person tells you about their thoughts or concerns, take time to confirm with them that you have understood what it is they are trying to tell you. Check back with them periodically, recapping on what has been said. Phrases such as 'Can I check that you mean …?' or 'What you have told me so far is …, have I got that right?' can help (Mannix, 2021, p. 283). Doing this both confirms that you have understood what has been said and that the person talking with you knows that you have this understanding.

It is important to support the person talking to you by remaining *curious* as they talk, this helps the person feel listened to (Mannix, 2021, p. 283). By asking curious questions as they talk, you can help and support their narrative to unfold; questions such as 'Would you tell me about …?' or 'I'd like to hear more about ...' can facilitate this. It enables you to appear open-minded about the conversation and meet as equals.

However, there may be times where someone may be uncertain how to start a conversation about a topic they are worried about. Their worry may stem from how the conversation may turn out, or they may be concerned about having things they feared confirmed to them. Leaving these thoughts in an unspoken state, however, may not be helpful and you can help facilitate a conversation by inviting the person into it.

First, remember: it is very easy if someone asks you a challenging question such as 'Am I going to die, nurse?' to brush off the request for a conversation with a straightforward platitude such as 'Of course not', or 'Don't be silly, we're here to make you better.' However, the fact someone has asked a tricky question such as this or 'Do you think I will get well enough to live again at home?' indicates that it is something they are concerned about and that they are looking for help talking through their concerns. As a student nurse you may not feel well qualified enough to give an answer to questions; however, you can help support an individual to share their concerns with you. You can also give assurance, that, where you don't know an answer to a question, there will be other members of the healthcare team who, with the patient's permission, you will be able to ask.

Responding to difficult questions with phrases such as 'Is there anything in particular that makes you ask that?' or, more generally, 'Tell me how have things been for you recently?' gives the person asking you the opportunity to tell you more about what is behind their concerns. It also shows them that you are interested in what they have to say and that you are inviting them to tell you more. Remember that you don't need to have the answers to any questions; by inviting the conversation to proceed, you are enabling them to share the burden of their concerns with you. You are providing a space for them to feel listened to.

In providing that space, don't be afraid to leave silences. It is very easy to try and fill gaps in a conversation by interjecting. Silence, however, allows the person who is discussing things that are challenging to reflect, pause and gather their thoughts before deciding how to move on with the conversation. If you find it difficult to hold a silence, you can try using open questions that reflect back components of what has just been said, 'You were saying that the results made you worried ...', 'So, you've felt like you have been getting worse for a while ...' and check your understanding of this, 'Have I got that right?' Bridging the silence like this can support a person to continue talking and show them that you are still engaged with what they are saying.

Don't be afraid to say that you don't have the answers or solutions to their concerns. The person you are listening to is unlikely to mind that, and will no doubt be grateful that you have spent time with them, listening. Seek their permission to ask their questions of others more senior to you in the team and give an assurance that you will get back to them. In doing this, you become a facilitator to finding a way forward with any concerns they may have and what matters to them in their future care; without you spending time listening, this may not have happened.

Responsibilities of a student nurse

As a student nurse it is important for you to ensure you are aware if someone has their wishes written down in the form of a DNACPR, ADRT or advance care plan, or establishing that an attorney is acting on a patient's behalf. You can do this by asking questions about this at your formal patient handovers, or by reading a patient's notes. Asking questions about all forms of advance planning can also help raise awareness of the importance of this for the people in your care.

In the case study at the start of this chapter, Kai had been asked by her uncle, Lei, about how he might start to plan for the things that may happen to him as his MND progresses.

Concept summary: motor neurone disease

Motor neurone disease (MND), also known as amyotrophic lateral sclerosis (ALS), is a neurodegenerative disease. It is currently without cure, with the average time between diagnosis and death being two to three years. It has a sudden onset, rapid progression and brings with it the potential for complex and disabling symptoms and care needs. The progression of symptoms and subsequent onset of disability are likely to occur over weeks and months rather than years. Because of the life-limiting, progressive nature of MND advance planning is vital in ensuring that potential future healthcare needs are discussed early in the course of the disease.

Reflecting back on the different components of planning for the end of life explored in this chapter, and the progressive nature of MND, we can start to think about which of these Kai may consider could be helpful to support her Uncle Lei in his planning.

Case study: Lei's planning for the end of life

Do not attempt cardiopulmonary resuscitation (DNAPCR)

It may be helpful for Lei have a discussion with his GP, or MND doctor or specialist nurse about the possible benefits and harms of attempting cardiopulmonary resuscitation in the event that his heart or breathing suddenly stops.

Advance decision to refuse treatment (ADRT)

There may be particular forms of treatment that Lei may wish not to have as his illness progresses and, if this was the case, he would need to ensure these are documented in an ADRT. Again, it is important for any treatments Lei thinks he may wish to refuse in the future to be discussed with a healthcare professional who has expertise in care of people with MND. This is important as they will be able to talk through with him the potential implications of stating that he wishes to refuse a specific form of treatment. In relation to MND, the kind of future treatments that may be discussed include the need for artificial feeding, should Lei lose the ability to swallow, or assisted ventilation should his respiratory muscles weaken to the point he needs external support.

Power of attorney

While he has mental capacity, Lei may wish to consider appointing an attorney to act on his behalf regarding his health and social care and his property and financial affairs should he lose mental capacity in the future. If Lei chooses to appoint one or more attorneys, then it is very helpful for them to know of the kind of choices Lei might make for himself which could be documented in an advance care plan.

(Continued)

(Continued)

Advance care plan

Given the complexity of symptoms and care needs that can be associated with the progression of MND there are many factors that Lei may wish to plan for in relation to what kind of care he may want, how that care may be delivered, where his care may be located and where he may wish to die. There may be additional considerations such as what alternative methods of communication he may wish to use if he loses the ability to speak, whether he may want alternative routes for nutrition should he lose the ability to swallow and whether he may wish to use assisted ventilation. You can see that there may be overlap with an ADRT here; however, the difference is that an ACP can help someone outline what they may want in terms of their future care. Conversely, an ADRT clearly details what treatments will be refused and in what circumstances that refusal will happen.

Assisted suicide and euthanasia

At the time of writing this book both **assisted suicide** and **euthanasia** are illegal in the United Kingdom. Parliamentary bills on assisted suicide and euthanasia are in the process of being discussed and debated through each of the devolved governments. Currently, any end of life planning cannot legally involve any planning for assisted suicide or euthanasia. Many people hold strong views on assisted suicide and euthanasia and it can be a polarising subject. Sometimes, requests to discuss this stem from other anxieties about the end of life, and it can be helpful to understand what is underpinning the person's thinking in relation to assisted suicide and euthanasia. This may lead to more general advance care planning conversations and the opportunity to discuss what dying might be like for them.

For more information on assisted suicide and euthanasia see: www.nhs.uk/conditions/euthanasia-and-assisted-suicide/

Chapter summary

This chapter has explored the idea of planning for the end of life. It started by focusing on the idea of what matters to people in life, moving to what might be important to someone as they approach the end of their life. The chapter has outlined the formal processes associated with planning for the end of life including DNACPR, ADRT and ACP and has explored ways in which you may help support people in talking about their future plans. The activities included in the chapter have invited you to reflect on the various aspects of end of life planning, and what you have experienced in clinical practice.

Further reading

Mannix, K (2021) *Listen: How to Find the Words for Tender Conversations.* London: HarperCollins.

We have referred to this book in this chapter, and recommend reading the entire book to help with all aspects of communication in relation to your practice. In relation to planning for the end of life, the chapters contained in the section 'Opening the box' (pp. 15–85) are particularly helpful, as is the section on 'Lessons in listening' (p. 167). Pages 282–285 contain a 'Style guide' for listening, with helpful phrases and prompts to use in conversations.

Rietjens, J, Korfage, I and Seymour, J (2021) Advance care planning, in Cherny, N, Fallon, M, Kaasa, S, Portenoy, R and Currow, D (eds), *Oxford Textbook of Palliative Medicine.* Oxford: Oxford University Press.

Chapter 31 summarises the evidence around advance care planning well from an international perspective.

Useful websites

www.nhs.uk/conditions/end-of-life-care/advance-decision-to-refuse-treatment/

NHS website exploring advance decisions to refuse treatment.

www.hospiceuk.org/our-campaigns/dying-matters/dying-matters-resources

These webpages are from Dying Matters, a campaign led by Hospice UK whose aim is *to create an open culture in which everyone is comfortable talking about death, dying and bereavement.* The resources section of the website includes leaflets on things to do before you die, talking to people affected by dementia about dying and talking to children about death and dying.

www.nhs.uk/conditions/social-care-and-support-guide/making-decisions-for-someone-else/mental-capacity-act/

NHS webpage providing information on the Mental Capacity Act.

www.mndassociation.org/

Website of the MNDA providing information and support for people affected by MND, their informal carers and health professionals.

The following webpages give information about power of attorney across the four nations of the UK:

England and Wales: **www.gov.uk/power-of-attorney**

Scotland: **www.publicguardian-scotland.gov.uk/power-of-attorney**

Northern Ireland: **www.nidirect.gov.uk/articles/managing-your-affairs-and-enduring-power-attorney**

www.resus.org.uk/respect

The website for the ReSPECT process which supports the creation of *personalised recommendations for a person's clinical care and treatment in a future emergency in which they are unable to make or express choices.*

www.resus.org.uk/

Information on all aspects of cardiopulmonary resuscitation.

www.rcn.org.uk/clinical-topics/end-of-life-care/covid-19-guidance-on-dnacpr-and-verification-of-death

Information from the Royal College of Nurses on DNACPR and verification of death in relation to Covid-19.

www.whatmattersconversations.org/

This website is produced by a group of independent charities, research organisations and health and social care bodies. The group is helping to drive a movement to encourage lifelong 'What matters' conversations, to get people talking about what is important to each of us and to improve end of life care planning.

Chapter 7 Families and carers

NMC Future Nurse: Standards of Proficiency for Registered Nurses

This chapter will address the following platforms and proficiencies:

Platform 3: Assessing needs and planning care

At the point of registration, the registered nurse will be able to:

3.14 identify and assess the needs of people and families for care at the end of life, including requirements for palliative care and decision making related to their treatment and care preferences

3.15 demonstrate the ability to work in partnership with people, families and carers to continuously monitor, evaluate and reassess the effectiveness of all agreed nursing care plans and care, sharing decision making and readjusting agreed goals, documenting progress and decisions made

Platform 4: Providing and evaluating care

At the point of registration, the registered nurse will be able to:

4.2 work in partnership with people to encourage shared decision making in order to support individuals, their families and carers to manage their own care when appropriate

4.9 demonstrate the knowledge and skills required to prioritise what is important to people and their families when providing evidence-based person-centred nursing care at end of life including the care of people who are dying, families, the deceased and the bereaved

Chapter aims

After reading this chapter, you will be able to:

- describe the role of family and informal carers of people at the end of life
- recognise the possible impact on carers of supporting someone at the end of their life
- understand how health and social care professionals can support carers when providing end of life care
- identify local and national organisations that have a role in supporting carers.

Introduction

Case study: Cary

Cary had always been close to her grandparents, Grace and Michael Fitzwilliam. While they lived an hour's drive away from her family home, she had seen them most weekends and often stayed with them during the school holidays. They enjoyed her company and had been incredibly proud of her successes at school, and never more so than when she announced to them that she had been offered a place to study nursing at university.

Cary's grandpa had worked in the manufacturing industry all his life, spending long hours at the factory a short walk from her grandparents' home. After he retired, he and her grandma had enjoyed many holidays together, their favourite trips being coach tours where they would get to meet new people; they enjoyed discovering new places.

As they got older they were less able to take holidays as her grandpa was becoming increasingly tired and breathless. Cary's grandma, who was increasingly frail herself, was doing more and more of the jobs around the home that her grandpa used to do. They'd always been quite traditional in their roles around the house, but the last time Cary had visited, as she'd arrived, her grandma was lugging the heavy lawnmower across the grass trying to cut it. It broke Cary's heart to see her elderly grandma struggling to do the jobs her grandpa used to do with ease.

Cary was determined to find out during her visit how things really were for her grandparents. So while her grandpa was settled watching football on the television, she made a cup of tea for her grandma and they sat in the kitchen and chatted …

Case study: Gethin

Gethin didn't know what to do. He was so exhausted he couldn't think that morning, but he had the two girls to get to school and then needed to deal with his work emails.

He'd been up four times overnight adjusting Caitlin's ventilation mask, and also knew that the community dietician would be arriving at some point – it was always difficult to predict just when – to talk to them both about the possibility of artificial feeding for Caitlin now her swallowing was getting worse. He felt like he'd managed his new caring role really well when Caitlin was first diagnosed with motor neurone disease eight months ago. But she had deteriorated so quickly that he felt he couldn't keep up with everything now: the equipment, the medicines, the number of healthcare workers who came to the house each day. He was just about managing his job and the girls, but he wasn't sure how much longer he'd be able to cope with it all. He gave a wry smile as he reflected back to a year ago when he thought being a working husband and dad more than filled his time.

The overarching aim of palliative care is to improve, through an holistic approach to care, the *quality of life of patients (adults and children) and their families and informal carers who are facing problems associated with life-threatening illness* (WHO, 2022).

The case studies above portray two different pictures of how someone may become an informal carer and describe some of the challenges that may occur with this role. In this chapter we explore in more detail this key component of palliative care, working with a patient's family and informal carers to understand their experiences and help support them both in their caring role and as people living alongside someone who is approaching the end of their life. We explore who we mean by 'families and informal carers' and will look at how these people are those who deliver care to individuals living with life-limiting conditions but can also be recipients of care themselves.

We will look at how this dual position means that a patient's family and informal carers can have significant support needs and how, as a nurse, you can help identify and provide this support throughout the end of life trajectory, including bereavement.

Who are carers?

Many of us have taken on a caring role at some point in our lives. This may have been for a short period of time caring for someone who was acutely unwell, or over a longer period for someone living with a long-term condition or life-limiting illness. It may be that these caring experiences influenced your decision to become a nurse.

As part of this chapter, it is important that we consider what we mean when we use the term 'carer', as it may mean different things to different people. A number of different definitions exist, but for the purposes of this chapter we have chosen to use the definition used by the NHS in England:

> *A carer is anyone, including children and adults, who looks after a family member, partner or friend who needs help because of their illness, frailty, disability, a mental health problem or an addiction and cannot cope without their support. The care they give is unpaid.*
>
> NHS England (2022)

One of the key components of the definition of 'carer' is that last point, that it is unpaid. It is this which differentiates people providing informal care, from those who have this as a formal job, with pay. Carers can come in many forms; we often talk of family members as key carers, but equally, neighbours, friends, community members, or work colleagues may take on the role. Many carers don't see themselves as such and can be surprised when they are called someone's carer. Often, caring occurs through an existing family relationship – for example, a husband caring for his wife after she has a stroke; a grown up daughter caring for her father who has dementia; a child caring for a parent with a long-term condition or disability.

Family and carers play a vital role in supporting people as they recover from an acute illness, a short period in hospital or as they live with a long-term condition. This support also extends to caring for someone as they approach the end of their life, whether following a very short illness, or one that has deteriorated over a number of years (Hardy, 2018). Carers are the individuals who, more than anyone else involved in care, enable people to live at home at the end of their lives. The following activity invites you to consider people who you have come across during clinical placements who may have been involved, informally, in people's care.

Activity 7.1   Reflection

Think back to one of your recent clinical placements and the patients and family members that you encountered there. Were you aware whether any family members were providing care for the patients you were looking after? If so, how did you know about this – that is, through conversations with the patient or their family, nursing or other clinical notes, nursing handover etc.?

There are no answers provided to this activity as it is based on your own observations.

Understanding if there are people supporting patients in your care, informally at home or elsewhere, is an important step to help you to appreciate the role they play in each patient's care. Carers are not always identified in practice (as you may have observed when you undertook Activity 7.1), but this identification is the important first step in assessing what support carers may benefit from.

Being an informal carer

You will come across people who are carers in all the settings where you have clinical placements. The role carers play as someone nears the end of their life, and to which we are referring here, may come at the end of a long period of caring. This may have started as a more minor role of support but may have subtly grown in involvement as a person becomes more ill and more dependent. This can result in the carer taking on increasingly complex aspects of care, often becoming an expert in what it takes to support the person at home (Flemming et al., 2019).

Throughout a life-limiting illness, patients and those who informally support them in their care have to manage their illness independently between their contacts with healthcare professionals (Hardy et al., 2014). This may be in between visits to hospital as an in-patient or out-patient or between visits from community-based nurses and other professionals. Carers take on many roles: these include the provision of physical care, household management, organisation of financial affairs and the adoption of roles which may previously have been undertaken by the ill person (Hardy et al., 2014). In many instances, if a person wishes to be cared for and die at home, the presence of an informal carer is essential in facilitating this to happen. However, becoming a carer may not be a specific choice made by an individual, but one that comes about through the relationship the individual has with the person – for example, as spouse, son, daughter or sibling. Caregiving is often seen as an expected extension of family relationships and, through these relationships, people may feel there is little option as to whether they undertake the role.

As a result, people who become carers may feel as if they have relinquished their relationship with the person they are caring for. The position of husband, wife, daughter may feel like it has vanished; instead they have become the person on whom they depend and without which an individual may not be able to remain at home.

Many carers talk of the stresses and strains associated with caring for someone, even when it is a role they have chosen and wish to do. Carers are often very committed to the care they provide, feel constantly responsible for the care that is received by their loved one (Hardy et al., 2014) and because of this may feel unable to take a break from their caring role. This may be because there is no one else available to take on this caring, or it may be that the individual's care needs are quite complex and those who could substitute for the carer may not have the knowledge and skills to manage the care.

The feeling of responsibility for care may not be relinquished when someone is admitted to hospital. The carer may feel a responsibility and need to visit regularly to ensure that the person is being cared for well and to advocate for them, particularly if the person themselves lacks mental capacity.

As a result of their enduring responsibilities, carers often become tired and worn out by their caring role. Sleep may be disrupted by needing to provide care during the night leading to exhaustion. Additionally, the ongoing responsibility and time devoted to caregiving can compromise opportunities people have available to do other things, even to take time for themselves. This can be further exacerbated if care is being provided alongside other roles. For example, it can be quite common for an adult child, for example, to be providing regular care for one or more of their parents while also having dependent children to look after at the same time. This kind of 'juggling' of care can impact on all aspects of the carer's life, their work, career plans, relationships, hobbies and social life.

For those carers who live with the person they care for, the impact of caring may be more profound, particularly if leaving the person alone is unfeasible, even for a short period of time. People may also have to adapt to a changing home environment. As the health of the individual deteriorates, increasing amounts of medical and supportive equipment may be required, and there may be an increase in the numbers of health and social care professionals who visit the home. The carer may experience a loss of privacy as the personal space of 'home' is changed into a medicalised environment and may feel pushed aside in a space that was theirs (Hardy et al., 2014).

Additionally, a person's carer may have ongoing health needs themselves. For example, a partner who cares for an older person may be living with one or more illnesses themselves which they need help and support with. There is a risk that carers may neglect their own health needs while caring for someone else, perceiving that their own health isn't as important as the care they need to provide. Being an older person caring for an older person can take an enormous toll on their physical and mental health. The following activity asks you to consider the impact of caring on those providing informal care.

Activity 7.2   Critical thinking

Re-read the two case studies at the beginning of the chapter and the section 'Being an informal carer' above and consider what the impact of being a carer might be for:

1.   Cary's grandma as she lives with her increasing frailty while trying to support and care for her breathless and ailing husband;
2.   Gethin as he juggles the increasing care needs that Caitlin has, alongside being a father to two young girls and his responsibilities to his job.

A suggested answer is provided at the end of the chapter.

You will have identified a broad range of potential impact of caring on Cary and Gethin in Activity 7.2. Understanding the impact of caring on someone with an informal caring role can then help you to identify areas in which support may be helpful to them.

Supporting a patient's family and carers

We have explored what we mean by the term 'carer', how people may become carers and some of the impacts there might be on an individual when they are a carer.

It is a key role of the nurse to support a patient's family members, including those who are informal carers. The proficiencies outlined at the start of the chapter highlight the key responsibilities including:

- having the ability to work in partnership with family and carers, sharing decision-making with them and planning and evaluating care;
- knowing how to prioritise what is important both to the patient and their family at the end of life and providing this care in a person-centred way.

This can feel like a daunting task as a student nurse. Depending on where your first clinical placements are during your education, it is likely that your early experiences of working alongside and supporting families and informal carers of people who are at the end of life will either be in the hospital setting or, if on a community-based placement, in people's own homes. You may also meet family carers if you are on placement in a nursing or residential home or hospice.

When you meet a patient and their carer/family in hospital, this may be at the end of a period of time in which both the patient and their carer have been trying to manage caring at home and to remain at home. It is worth bearing in mind that while as health professionals we may see the difference between someone being cared for at home and in hospital as being quite distinct, for patients and their carers the two may be much more linked. The role of caring doesn't stop at the point someone is admitted, it may just take on a different form, with a carer still feeling responsibility as the patient's advocate, ensuring that they are well looked after; this can also be the case when a person is first admitted to a nursing or residential care home. As a nurse it is important that you recognise the role that a carer plays at home. When a patient is admitted into a formal care environment, the knowledge about the patient that they hold is important for continuity of the patient's care; they will also need to be assured that the person will be well cared for while they are there.

Therefore, the setting in which you first meet a patient and their family and informal carers will guide the way you develop your relationship and support with them. In people's own homes, you are the patient's guest and will work around how they have set up their home and care routines. Your visits are likely to be relatively short in length and, while they may increase in frequency towards the end of life, there may equally be an extended period of time between visits. As a result, it may feel like it is quite difficult to get to know people well enough to be able to feel you can work in partnership with them and understand what is important to them to be able to prioritise this. However, working with people in their own homes gives you a unique insight into how things are for people, how they are coping, what resources they have to help them manage caring, such as whether they are working, have other dependents reliant on them and what the physical space is for equipment. This is an insight that you wouldn't have access to in the same way if the person was being cared for in hospital or care home. It can really help to facilitate your broader understanding about an individual, help you work out what is important to them and give you cues for conversations to enable you to learn more about a person.

Scenario: Mr and Mrs Fitzwilliam

You are working on a community nursing placement, visiting patients in their own homes. One of your visits takes you to the home of Mr and Mrs Fitzwilliam, an elderly couple who, you have been told, are starting to 'struggle to cope' at home. Michael Fitzwilliam, who receives twice-weekly visits from the district nursing team to dress his longstanding leg ulcer, has increasingly been breathless and having difficulty walking, while his wife Grace is becoming very frail. You have the chance to chat to Grace while Michael's ulcer is being dressed. Grace tells you that she is having to provide more and more care for Michael, including helping him to get washed and dressed and give him his medications. Grace then confesses that she is worrying about how she will manage as she sees Michael getting worse. She knows she is struggling but doesn't want him to go into care. She tells you that their granddaughter, who is a student nurse like you, visited yesterday. Grace goes on to say that she didn't want to share her concerns with Cary, as she knew she would worry, and she and the rest of the family live too far away to help.

Having thought about the impact of being an informal carer for someone in the previous activity, the next activity invites you to think about what might be important for a carer in their caring role.

Activity 7.3   Critical thinking

From the scenario above, think about some of the ways you could start to understand what is important to Grace, as Michael's wife and carer, along with what worries her.

Outline answers to guide your thinking in relation to this activity are provided at the end of the chapter.

Having considered what might be important to someone as an informal carer in their own home in Activity 7.3, let us now consider the role of an informal carer in a formal healthcare setting. In a hospital, for example, the patient and their family/informal carers are in 'your' environment (even if this might still feel a bit alien to you at times). As a result, they may feel less comfortable; be uncertain as to where things are; have limited understanding of the processes and procedures that are happening around them (which may feel very familiar to you) and the time frame in which things happen (either slow or fast); and may also have worries as to whether care will be given in the way it would have been at home. They may also feel stressed and tired following a period of trying to 'manage' at home and, perhaps because of a deterioration or exacerbation in the patient's condition, being less able recently to do this. An admission can also be a planned one, for a particular procedure or intervention.

As a patient is admitted into hospital one of your primary roles is to provide reassurance and support to them and their family and carers. Taking time to ensure they are introduced to you and other members of the healthcare team, have a sense of what might occur in the next few hours and days (where it is known) and being given information on the ward layout, facilities for visitors and how to contact the ward can all help contribute to a sense of feeling supported and cared for. It is important to involve carers, with the patient's permission, in all of these discussions and, additionally, to ask the carer how involved they may want to be in someone's care, particularly if the person who is unwell is unable to communicate this for themselves. It is worth remembering that many carers develop a high-level of expertise and tacit knowledge through their time as carers, so are often well placed to be the patient's advocate.

Information valued by carers

The support you provide for carers can be enhanced by having an understanding of the kind of information carers say is helpful to know. Drawing on qualitative research which explores, from carers' perspectives, what helps and hinders them in their role, it is possible to develop an understanding as to what carers' needs are and how you might be able to support them.

A systematic review of qualitative research synthesised 34 papers exploring the information needs of over 900 carers providing care for someone with an advanced life-limiting condition. The papers included in the review interviewed carers in the USA, UK, Canada and Australia, 75 per cent of whom were female. Just over half (58 per cent) of the carers in the included studies were married to the person they were caring for. Care was being provided for people with a wide range of advanced illnesses including cancer, chronic obstructive pulmonary disease, neurodegenerative conditions, renal disease, heart failure and dementia (Flemming et al., 2019).

The findings of the review identified key information needs of carers which spanned across the trajectory of a patient's illness. Carers identified their information needs changed over the course of the illness (no matter what its type).

Carers value information from the point at which the diagnosis of an advanced life-limiting illness is made to ensure they have understanding of what to expect. Carers commonly want to know about the likely course a disease can take so that they have a sense of what might happen, and that important planning and conversations can take place.

Caring for someone can be a complex role, requiring a number of skills. The review discussed the kind of information and education that can help carers prepare for the role and support them through it. Ideally, information is given as early as possible, allowing carers time to think it through and to ask any questions that may arise. Overall, information that addresses the physical tasks of caring for someone was seen as the most important.

Carers often feel considerable responsibility for managing symptoms and administering medications. Being able to understand and manage patients' symptoms really helped carers to have confidence to continue their caring role at home. Having the knowledge to recognise symptoms and know how to manage them was important. It was seen as preferable to have this knowledge in advance of symptoms occurring, rather than trying to work out what to do during an emergency situation.

If a patient is on a lot of medication or the medication regimen is complex, this can lead to a greater sense of a burden of care for carers and make them feel more anxious about what they are doing. However, in response, many carers develop techniques to help them monitor, record and report medicines administration, keeping records for themselves. They also show these reports to visiting health professionals in order to get reassurance that they are 'doing the right thing'. Having high-quality, relevant information can be really useful; when carers feel well informed, they tend to have increased confidence in decisions around managing medicines and other aspects of care.

Being given information ahead of things happening is important to carers. The idea of 'hoping for the best but planning for the worst' gives confidence in both what to expect and how they will deal with it. This is particularly the case for acute exacerbations of illness such as severe episodes of breathlessness; when information on managing acute events is given to carers they feel more confident in their ability to cope with the situations as they unfold.

As a patient's disease progresses, carers can welcome information on the processes around dying. It is seen as crucial to carers to know what to expect during the dying phase as this helps them overcome and dispel fears as to what they think might happen.

Studies that involve bereaved carers have highlighted information carers would have found helpful in preparation for bereavement. Some of the information that carers find useful and particularly when given before death, includes detail on the very practical aspects in the period immediately following a person's death, such as funeral planning, registration of death and management of finances. These studies also show how carers' experiences of caring, both good and bad, stay with them and can shape how their bereavement progresses.

Understanding what information is key to a carer being able to successfully carry out their role is important; the next activity invites you to consider this further.

Activity 7.4   Critical thinking

Looking back to Gethin's case at the start of the chapter, consider how the information presented above on carers' information needs might help you think through information that might be helpful to Gethin in relation to:

- the rapid trajectory of Caitlin's illness
- Caitlin's respiratory support and other possible interventions
- planning for the future.

Outline answers to guide your thinking in relation to this activity are provided at the end of the chapter.

Activity 7.4 has helped you to focus on what information may be helpful to someone in a caring role in the context of one particular scenario. The following section discusses research which has explored carers' information needs more broadly.

What carers say helps them

There are a number of approaches to supporting carers that carers themselves have reported as being really helpful in their caring role (Flemming et al., 2019):

1. *The importance of professional relationships*

   The quality of the relationship between health professionals (either individually or as part of a team) and the carer can be really influential on a carer's perception of their caring experience. When carers perceive they have positive relationships with the healthcare professionals supporting them, this really helps to relieve the burden of caring.

2. *Proactive advice and support*

   In the section above we saw how helpful it was when information is given in advance of things happening. Proactive advice and help from health professionals, anticipating both patients' and carers' needs, really adds to a sense of perceived support by carers. Regular communication and information-giving, through phone contact or quick 'check-ins', alongside more formal planned meetings can be particularly valued.

   There are many ways in which proactive advice can occur – for instance, health professionals anticipating when pain control may be needed; spotting when there may be a need for a carer to have some respite; support and guidance for decision-making around aspects of care; making contact without prompting.

3. *Placing the whole family at the centre of care*

   Putting the family rather than the individual patient at the centre of care is highly valued by carers. This can be achieved by giving time to answer questions, checking understanding and by giving choice as to how information is communicated with people. Good communication of information underpins the sense of trust that carers have in health professionals.

Overall, positive relationships with health professionals, facilitated through timely access, compassionate communication and proactive support, are highly valued by carers and help to relieve the burden of caring.

When care is being provided at the end of life

There will be times when you will be involved in caring for a patient towards the very end of their life. This may be in the patient's own home, in hospital or a care home, or hospice. Your focus of care at this point continues to be one which places the whole family at the centre of care, ensuring that care is personalised to the patient's wishes.

It is likely that the person who has provided most of the patient's care in the last days, weeks and perhaps months of life remains with the person during the last days of life; most probably this will be a close family member of the person who is dying. The individual concerned may want at this point to relinquish their more formal role of caring and resume being the dying person's spouse, son, daughter, mother, father, brother or sister etc. …

When someone is dying it can feel daunting as a student nurse walking into a hospital room, or entering a home, knowing that there are a number of family members who may look to you for cues as to what is happening as the patient is dying. They may be fearful of deterioration, and seek explanations around particular symptoms or sounds that the person is experiencing or making. Have confidence in your ability to be alongside those family members, be honest if you are not sure, but reassure them that you will ask their question to a more senior nurse.

Tools for practice: 'What matters' to you conversations

It is helpful to have some prompts to support you in having conversations with patients and family members when it may feel awkward or difficult to do so. A useful framework for conversations called the 'What matters' to you 'how to' guide (Figure 7.1) has been developed by collaboration between patients, professionals and healthcare organisations. Its use in practice has been piloted with a variety of health professionals. The guide was developed by Turner and Millington-Sanders (2022) on behalf of the End of Life Care Partners Think Tank (2021). The Think Tank is a group of independent charities, research organisations and health and social care bodies who are helping to drive a movement to encourage 'What matters' conversations. We discussed more about planning for care at the end of life in Chapter 6.

WHAT MATTERS TO YOU CONVERSATIONS

A "how to" guide

WHY?

- ○ Improves communication, human connection and shows others we care
- ○ We often learn something new
- ○ Avoids our personal judgements
- ○ Gives people permission & opportunity to be honest about what matters most to them
- ○ Useful for in-depth or focused conversations

BEFORE

- ○ Is there someone else you should be involving?
- ○ Do they have any communication or information needs?
- ○ Check it's the right time and place for the person and you

---

(?) ASK

- ○ Be curious, be kind, be present.
- ○ Example of open questions: 'what matters most to you right now/today/in the future?', 'what's worrying you most?', 'what/who is most important to you?', 'how can I best support you?', "what makes a good/bad day for you?', is there anything I can do to make things better?', 'is there 'anything else you think I should know?'

↓

◁》 LISTEN

- ○ Show you're listening – verbal and non-verbal affirmation
- ○ Reflect back what you've heard
- ○ Listen for cues - follow up with questions if clarity needed

↓

⊘ DO

- ○ Active listening = doing
- ○ Explore quick wins and discuss what may need more planning
- ○ Mutually agree on actions or signposting
- ○ Sometimes it's not 'doable' – but explain why and explore further what it is that really matters most and what is possible

AFTER

- ○ Record the conversation (as appropriate)
- ○ Follow up on agreed actions
- ○ Reflect on your learning

Figure 7.1 'What matters' to you conversation 'how to' guide

Activity 7.5 invites you to consider the information provided in the 'how to' guide in the context of your clinical practice.

Activity 7.5 Reflection

Read the 'how to' guide to in Figure 7.1.

1. Think about a recent conversation you have had with a patient and their family or carer.
2. Consider whether you used an 'Ask', 'Listen', 'Do' approach to the conversation.
3. Think about what aspects of the conversation went well and where areas for improvement could be.

There are no answers provided to this activity as it is based on your own thoughts.

Having a prompt such as the 'how to' guide can help support you and give you confidence in your conversations with a patient and their family. Often when a person is nearing the end of their life, there may be multiple family members who wish to visit and you may need to speak with. In these instances, it is helpful to identify among these people who it is who will be the main point of contact for updates and information who can then cascade this information to other family members or friends. This is often the person who has been the main carer prior to someone getting admitted to hospital or becoming more unwell, but, at times, this role may be taken on by someone else.

There is a lot you can do as a student nurse to help support a patient's family and carers towards the end of life. It may feel to you as if your role is quite peripheral at such a crucial time in life. However, a patient's family will gain much comfort and confidence from your presence, and, as a student nurse, you may be in a position to be alongside a family more than other members of the healthcare team. By using the key components of 'Ask', 'Listen', 'Do' detailed in the 'how to' guide in your interactions with family members, and seeking advice from more experienced colleagues if you feel unsure, you will be well placed to provide positive support to people, which may well be remembered by them for a long time to come. Doing this will support you to develop the knowledge and skills required as a registered nurse.

Chapter summary

This chapter has explored the role of family and informal carers of people at the end of life. It has sought to identify who carers are and the way in which they may become a carer. It has examined the impact that caring can have on an individual, particularly when they are supporting someone through an advanced life-limiting illness. It has provided guidance as to the kinds of information carers find valuable to know. It also provides suggestions as to how you can support family members and carers as someone close to them nears the end of their life. Throughout the chapter, we have placed particular emphasis on the importance of understanding 'what matters' to patients, their family and carers at the final stage of someone's life, and how you, as a student nurse, can elicit and act on this.

Activities: brief outline answers

Activity 7.2   Critical thinking (page 124)

Cary's grandma may face a number of significant challenges as she takes on the role of carer for her husband, many of which will be related to her age and frailty. These may include: her own health being impacted by the additional strain of managing an increasing number of physical household tasks, lack of sleep and rest; the restrictions on her ability to care for her husband in the way she might like to because of her frailty; the psychological stress of 'not managing' in the way she might like to; potential difficulties of day-to-day support from the wider family because they live some distance away; reduced ability to attend appointments and check-ups for herself due to her caring role; anticipatory grief in relation to her husband's death.

Gethin has a significant number of different roles to 'juggle' while caring for Caitlin. He has rapidly had to take on an increasingly complex and demanding caring role for Caitlin due to the speed of her deterioration. This is likely to impact on Gethin in a number of ways including: lack of sleep, reduced ability to undertake his work responsibilities, predominantly sole responsibility for caring for his children and their support needs; increasing time coordinating hospital appointments and care visits; increasing responsibility for managing symptoms, medication regimes and medical equipment; anticipatory grief in relation to Caitlin's death.

Activity 7.3   Critical thinking (page 126)

You can start to understand what is important to Grace by listening with the aim of understanding her concerns and experiences. In the scenario, Grace provides a number of preliminary cues as to what is important to her and also that concern her:

*   her willingness to provide care for Michael
*   her wish that she would like him to stay at home with her
*   a desire not to worry her wider family with her concerns.

Grace also highlights some things that are worrying her:

*   Michael's visible deterioration
*   her ability to manage the increasing responsibility of caring for Michael given her own health
*   the distance that her family are from her and therefore their ability to help if things get more difficult.

Activity 7.4   Critical thinking (page 128)

*   *The rapid trajectory of Caitlin's illness*

    Gethin may benefit from understanding more about what is coming next in the course of Caitlin's illness, helping him to both anticipate and plan for these. In diseases where decline can happen very quickly over weeks or months, then carers can often feel as if they can't keep up. Knowing what to expect, as far as it possible to say, can give carers more of a sense of control.

*   *Caitlin's respiratory support and other possible interventions*

    Planning for future exacerbations of breathlessness and weakening respiratory muscles may help Gethin manage acute events when they arise. It is important to also explore less anticipated events. Caitlin's swallowing is weakening, so episodes of choking may be likely. Knowing that this is a possibility and strategies to manage if it does occur can be helpful in instilling a sense of control, although need to be carefully communicated to avoid causing additional anxiety about their situation.

- *Planning for the future*

  Caitlin has deteriorated very quickly. Having someone speak with both Gethin and Caitlin about her future care needs, what treatments and interventions she may or may not want – for example, artificial feeding, permanent ventilation, intravenous antibiotics, how to support their children and her preferred place for care and death – can ensure there are plans in place as situations arise. These may adapt and change; however, the initial thinking has been discussed and documented.

Further reading

Bunting, M (2021) *Labours of Love: The Crisis of Care.* London: Granta.

In this book Madeleine Bunting writes of first-hand accounts of caring, including a history of caring and the language associated with it. It provides a vital overview of the landscape of care in the UK.

Ewing, G, Austin, L, Diffin, J and Grande, G (2015) Developing a person-centred approach to carer assessment and support. *British Journal of Community Nursing,* 20(12), 580–584.

In this paper the authors discuss how community nurses play an important role in providing palliative care and support for patients and carers at home. They describe the development of a tool called the Carer Support Needs Assessment Tool (CSNAT) which provides practitioners with an evidence-based tool to use with carers in palliative home care. The CSNAT uses a person-centred approach, with the process of carer assessment and support being facilitated by practitioners while being carer-led.

The Reluctant Carer (2022) *The Reluctant Carer: Dispatches from the End of Life.* London: Picador.

The Reluctant Carer is a funny, honest and moving account of one individual's experiences of moving back home to help out his elderly parents during a crisis and finding that he is there to stay as their carer.

Useful websites

General support for carers

www.ageuk.org.uk/services/in-your-area/carers-support/

Age UK: *Caring for an older person can be a rewarding but challenging job. Our local Age UKs offer much-needed practical and emotional support to unpaid carers and provide opportunities for respite from caring duties.*

www.carersuk.org/home

Carers UK: *The UK's only charity for carers, Carers UK is both a supportive community and a movement for change for people who are providing care for others.*

www.nhs.uk/conditions/social-care-and-support-guide/support-and-benefits-for-carers/carer-breaks-and-respite-care/

NHS England: Carers' breaks and respite care – respite care means taking a break from caring, while the person being cared for is looked after by someone else.

www.whatmattersconversations.org/

End of life Think Tank (2021) The webpages for 'What matters' conversations that we discussed in the chapter.

Specific carer support for people near the end of life

www.hospiceuk.org/information-and-support/your-guide-hospice-and-end-life-care/support-carers/caring-someone-home#content-menu-737

Hospice UK: *Caring for someone who is at the end of their life at home can be rewarding, but also very challenging. This page has advice on where to get support and how to take care of yourself if you are a carer.*

www.mariecurie.org.uk/help/support/being-there

Marie Curie: *Caring for a friend or family member with a terminal illness can be both rewarding and challenging. Marie Curie's information can help carers know what to expect – from day-to-day caring to looking after their own needs.*

Chapter 8 Research and evidence-based practice in palliative and end of life care

Chapter aims

After reading this chapter, you will be able to:

- understand what we mean by evidence-based practice
- explain why it is important that we have an evidence base for palliative and end of life care
- appreciate some of the challenges associated with conducting research with people nearing the end of life
- give examples of the nurse's role in finding, appraising and using evidence to inform patient care and relate this to your own practice
- be aware of the role of pre-appraised evidence in clinical decision-making.

Introduction

Case study: Stephan

Stephan is lying in bed pondering something he has been asked about. A research nurse came and spoke with him today offering him the opportunity to be involved in a research study of a drug that might help relieve one of the symptoms that is troubling him at the moment. He's really keen to take part, thinking it might help both him and also others with his illness, but he's worried about whether it is worth it. After all, he is dying …

This chapter presents the idea that research is important for palliative care and that this research forms the 'evidence base' on which you should base your nursing practice. What we want you to remember is that, for research to happen, people need to consent and give their time to take part in it. For Stephan, this clearly will impact on the time he has left to live, and the chapter will explore some of the reasons why people agree to take part in research at the end of their lives and why it is important that we continue to ask them to. As a nurse, you need to be able to find research evidence, be able to read and understand this, and communicate about it with patients and families. You will also be involved in research in other ways; this may include contributing to recruiting people to research studies, having a role where research is the main focus of your work, such as in research nursing, participating in research prioritisation exercises (where nurses and other people suggest where there are gaps in the evidence base and that research should be undertaken), or becoming a researcher yourself and establishing and leading research studies.

This chapter will explore with you why research is important and its role within palliative care. We will discuss the role of research in palliative care, what we mean by evidence-based practice and how this relates to research. We will briefly examine different types of evidence that inform practice, before focusing on research where we will specifically consider qualitative and quantitative research and specific types of reviews of research called 'systematic reviews'. The chapter will then discuss how we know what questions to ask in palliative care research. Finally, the chapter will guide you through the fundamentals of using research to inform your practice.

Our focus in this chapter is specifically on research and evidence as it relates to palliative and end of life care. As evidence-based practice is fundamental to *all* of your nursing practice, we encourage you to also read the other texts in this series which specifically address research and evidence-based practice in more depth than we have scope to cover here.

Research and evidence-based practice

Let's start with considering why research and other evidence might be important to you as a nurse. First, the Future Nurse Standards (NMC, 2018) require that you understand evidence-based practice and research and know how to apply it to your clinical practice; some of these proficiencies are outlined at the start of the chapter. The learning you undertake that enables you to meet these standards will place you in a strong position to support patients by delivering high-quality, effective and compassionate care that is also safe.

You may think using research to inform nursing practice is something relatively new; this is not quite the case! Florence Nightingale is viewed as one of the first nurses who sought to base her practice, and the practice of others, on research in order to improve patient outcomes. Nightingale developed the use of statistics to predict mortality. Through applying these data to nursing practice in field hospitals she demonstrated that most deaths in the Crimean War were not from battle injuries but from infection, and through her actions in changing infection prevention and control practices (as they would now be known), reduced mortality from infection by up to 99 per cent. Therefore, Nightingale did just what you are being asked to do today – used research findings to inform the care delivered to patients. Your role as a graduate nurse will be to convey complex information and ultimately to lead and develop nursing practice. Nightingale believed that the role of nurses was key to implementing improvements in healthcare and this remains the case 200 years later (Pattison et al., 2021).

Without having and using research to inform nursing practice, we know that aspects of care which intuitively may seem like the right thing to do can cause harm. It is only by evaluating care interventions and treatments using rigorous research methods that we can establish whether what intuitively seems like a good idea, based on relevant science, actually is. Similarly, we can only really understand what it is like to live with or through a particular illness or receive a type of treatment or care by asking people with the experience of doing just that, through research. There are different types of research methods that are used to evaluate nursing and healthcare; which type of method is used depends on the question that is being asked – we will explore these later in the chapter.

As you will know from learning about evidence-based nursing in your programme and through other reading, evidence-based practice involves more than just applying research evidence. It involves exploring what the patient's views are, considering available resources and incorporating expertise as part of any decision-making. It also involves communicating with people about the reasons for care and interventions, and we will explore this further later in this chapter. Research evidence is often summarised into guidelines; these are usually your first point of call in understanding the evidence in relation to a particular subject. Guidelines are developed through rigorous processes – for example, by the National Institute for Health and Care Excellence (NICE) – and are important and influential in practice. The focus of this chapter, however, is the production of research and how to find and appraise it in relation to palliative care.

For all the reasons outlined above, research is as important in palliative and end of life care as it is in any other healthcare discipline. We need robust research to be undertaken to ensure that we know that the care and treatment we provide for any person – but particularly those people at the end of life – is effective, relevant and appropriate. Each individual is different in their end of life care needs and what works best for them may not work for others. Within that, however, we need to know that 'what works best for them' is safe and effective.

What can be considered challenging in palliative care research, however, is the idea of people taking part in research at the end of their life. This brings us back to Stephan's conundrum …

Activity 8.1 Critical thinking

Stephan is nearing the end of his life, with possibly three months to live. He has had bone cancer for just over a year, which is causing him pain and, increasingly, fatigue. He has the opportunity to take part in a drug trial of new pain-relieving medication that may help manage his pain better.

Re-read the case study at the beginning of the chapter and answer the following questions which require you to consider your own views.

1.   Should people nearing the end of life be asked to take part in research?
2.   List three reasons why people might want to take part in a research study near the end of their life and three reasons why they might not.

Make some notes of your answers.

We have not provided answers to these questions as they are your own thoughts on these issues, but we will discuss these issues throughout the chapter.

Activity 8.1 asked to you consider your own views on involving people who are approaching the end of life in research, and reasons as to why they might want to participate. We believe that it is important to give people the choice to participate in research, so that they can make decisions based on what is right for them. Not offering people the choice could be viewed as paternalism and people can also view this as another threat to their autonomy.

Palliative care research conducted in the UK is some of the best in the world, and the results of these endeavours help to develop both the quality of the care that people receive and how palliative and end of life services are developed and run (Higginson, 2016). Despite its importance, the funding available for palliative care research is very limited when compared with research on the prevention and possible cure of life-limiting conditions. For example, less than 0.7 per cent of the £500 million spent on cancer research is allocated to palliative care (National Cancer Research Institute, 2015), with funding for non-cancer conditions likely to be even less. Therefore, despite the importance of research in palliative care, a robust evidence base can sometimes be lacking.

The relationship between research and evidence-based practice

'Evidence-based practice', or EBP, is the term given to using research to help inform your clinical practice. The aim of EBP is to try to reduce our uncertainty in clinical decision-making by incorporating appropriate, relevant and current research evidence into the decisions you make in clinical practice (Flemming, 2008) alongside other sources of information (including patient preference, available resources and clinical expertise). EBP began with the development of evidence-based medicine (EBM) in the early 1990s (Sackett et al., 1997) and has become a key component of both nursing education and practice.

What constitutes 'best evidence' to support your clinical practice is dependent on the type of clinical question or uncertainty you are wanting to answer and also the quality of the research you identify.

There are two main broad approaches to research (sometimes also referred to as research paradigms), qualitative and quantitative, and we explore each of these in turn below.

Qualitative research

Qualitative research is a type of research that is particularly good at exploring people's views and experience of particular aspects of their care, their illness, their treatment, the services they receive etc. As a result, it is a highly relevant research methodology for palliative care. A qualitative approach can help determine what health professionals' views or experiences of their roles and work are. It can also help explore 'what', 'how' and 'why' interventions do (or don't) work (Harris et al., 2018). Some of the different qualitative approaches used in nursing research include grounded theory, phenomenology, ethnography and case studies. The data collection methods used in qualitative research include in-depth interviews, focus groups, observations and stories in the form of diaries or other documents (Morley and Cathala, 2019). You can see an example of a qualitative study in palliative care in the box below.

Research summary: example of a qualitative study

Gerber, K, Hayes, B and Bryant, C (2019) 'It all depends!': a qualitative study of preferences for place of care and place of death in terminally ill patients and their family caregivers. *Palliative Medicine*, 33(7): 802–811.

Focus of the research: To understand how people who live with life-limiting conditions and their family caregivers make decisions about their preferred place of care and where they would like to die.

In this research, interviews were conducted with people with a life-limiting illness, thought to be in the last year of life, and carers to determine the decision-making process that patients and family caregivers use to develop their preferences around place of care and place of death.

The findings showed that people's preferences for place of care and death were shaped by the uncertainty of living with, or caring for someone with, a life-limiting illness. While, overall, home was the preferred place of care and was the place where people wanted to die, people also expressed uncertainty about it, as they were concerned about being a burden and carers were worried whether they would be able to cope with the demands of caring. If these concerns became significant, then it was felt that home was no longer a safe place to be cared for in, or to die.

People's views of hospital and other forms of institutional care were very much dependent on their prior experiences of these settings and what their family and friends thought of them, as well as representation in the media about such institutions.

Quantitative research

Quantitative research methods seek to measure and evaluate the effectiveness of healthcare interventions, often through randomised controlled trials (RCTs) and other forms of quantitative methods such as cohort studies, case control studies and economic evaluations. RCTs are the most appropriate research design for evaluating the effectiveness of clinical treatments, or interventions, and help to determine 'what works' in healthcare – for example, 'What effect does using treatment A or treatment B have on a particular outcome or outcomes?'

RCTs are important in addressing some of the clinical uncertainty we have in palliative care nursing as they are the best research design to answer questions which contain uncertainty around which treatment might be the best to try. This is a question of effectiveness, and nurses frequently ask questions of this nature (Nelson, 2011).

There are, however, challenges to conducting randomised controlled trials in palliative care, including the recruitment of participants into a trial. An RCT needs to have enough people recruited into it to be able to demonstrate that the difference between the treatments being compared is due to the intervention itself and not just due to chance. What this number is depends on both the treatment/intervention being studied and the outcomes that are being looked for – therefore it varies between research studies. Getting enough people recruited into palliative care clinical trials can be challenging due to how ill people may be at the point of recruitment. However, this challenge does not mean that RCTs aren't appropriate and relevant to palliative care, just that they need to be designed well, considering and planning for the ethical issues that relate to undertaking research with people who are vulnerable.

Research summary: example of a randomised controlled trial

Porter, L, Steel, J, Fairclough, T, LeBlanc,T, Bull, J et al. (2021) Caregiver-guided pain coping skills training for patients with advanced cancer: results from a randomised clinical trial. *Palliative Medicine*, 35(5): 952–961.

Question: Does training family carers to support people living with advanced cancer with their pain increase caregiver confidence and satisfaction and reduce caregiving strain?

This study sought to determine whether training carers of people living with advanced cancer pain would help improve the experience of caregiving in terms of satisfaction and confidence as well as improving the patient's pain.

In the RCT carers and the person they were caring for (a 'dyad') were randomised to either receive a pain education (the control group) or pain education plus pain coping skills training (the intervention group).

The findings showed that, compared to those in the control group, carers in the intervention group reported significant increases in caregiving satisfaction and decreased anxiety. In both groups carers reported improvements in self-efficacy, and patients reported improvements in self-efficacy, pain severity and interference, and psychological distress. As a result of the RCT we know that providing structured education and pain coping skills training may benefit patients and carers facing advanced cancer.

Systematic reviews

One of the ways we can overcome the problem of small numbers of people being recruited to clinical trials, or of other small research studies, is to review all the studies undertaken on a particular topic and bring them together in a systematic way – something known as a systematic review. Systematic reviews provide summaries of research-based knowledge on a specific topic, by using rigorous methods for searching and finding research, appraisal of the methodological strengths and limitations of the research, extracting data from the studies and combining these together through a process called 'synthesis'. Systematic reviews are really useful as, done well, all the high-quality research in a particular area is brought together in one place and distilled down to a small number of findings and recommendations – great for busy nurses to use!

Systematic reviews can be of quantitative or qualitative research; when only qualitative research is included in a systematic review the review is commonly called a qualitative evidence synthesis.

Activity 8.2   Evidence-based practice and research

Thinking back to Stephan's case study, research from which type of research paradigm would be best able to answer the following questions:

1.   What is the most effective form of analgesia to treat Stephan's bone pain?
2.   What do people living with life-limiting illnesses think about taking part in research?

Answers are provided at the end of the chapter.

How do researchers know what research questions to ask in palliative care?

We have explored some of the difficulties of undertaking research in relation to palliative and end of life care such as the small amount of funding available, the challenges of recruiting people into research studies and some of the concerns that arise from that, and you have tested your knowledge of different research paradigms in Activity 8.2. But how do researchers even know what is a good research question to answer, given these challenges around resource and recruitment to research? Given the obstacles in the way, it is vital that researchers are asking important questions that require answering – so how do they know this?

Often research questions will arise out of clinical uncertainty – that is, things we are uncertain about in our practice. As undergraduate nurses you probably won't have the scope or resources to undertake or 'do' research, but you can try to find research that other people have done to try to resolve that uncertainty – in other words, you can 'use' research other people have done. Later in this chapter we will explore how you can go about finding and using research in your practice.

One way that clinical uncertainty can be turned into research questions is through a 'research prioritisation exercise'. Bringing together clinicians, patients and carers to discuss research priorities is key as it enables all those affected to jointly discuss areas of clinical uncertainty and, in doing so, enables plans and priorities for future research to be identified. The James Lind Alliance set up the Palliative and end of life care Priority Setting Partnership (PeolcPSP) (James Lind Alliance, 2021). This involved over 1,400 people in the last years of life, current and former carers, health and social care professionals and organisations working together to determine the key unanswered questions for end of life care. The exercise resulted in key research questions being identified, many of which have attracted research funding enabling them to be answered.

Using research to inform your practice

What is key to any research is that it doesn't stop with the publication of a journal paper, but that it is used in practice; this is where you come in! As mentioned earlier in the chapter, the Future Nurse Standards (NMC, 2018) require that you understand research and know how to apply it to your nursing practice. We have also explored some of the reasons why this might be important. Let's look now at how using research to inform your practice might help you to support Stephan.

Activity 8.3   Evidence-based practice and research

While you are supporting Stephan with his daily wash, he starts to talk to you about the conversation he had with the research nurse. He says he is really interested in taking part in the research project, but wonders what other patients in his situation think as he has no experience of this. He is also worried about what his partner Michael may think about him using up some of the valuable time he has left in life to take part in research.

You say to him that you don't have much experience of this either but will do some finding out and get back to him tomorrow.

Think about how you might go about answering Stephan's question.

There are no definitive answers provided to this question as it is your own thoughts on this issue; however, some suggestions are provided at the end of the chapter.

Stephan has asked you a very common question: 'How do others in my situation feel about this?' You may have considered a range of ways of answering this in Activity 8.3, and this is an example of a clinical uncertainty. When patients are in new, uncertain and possibly anxiety-provoking situations they often want to know how others have felt about or managed that situation. As you gain more experience as a nurse you will be increasingly able to use the clinical expertise (knowledge) you have acquired to help answer patients' questions. That doesn't mean that you will always have the answers, or that your knowledge is based on up to date evidence, and it is important to develop the skills to draw on the broader evidence base to help support your patients in their decision-making.

So, how might you go about answering Stephan's question and finding out how other people who have taken part in research near the end of the lives have felt about this? One way would be to look to see if any research has been undertaken. This begins the process of EBP, the aim of which is to use best available research evidence to support you in your clinical decision-making.

There are other books in the Sage Transforming Nursing Practice series that explore the process of evidence-based practice in more detail. We have listed these in the

Further reading section and we would urge you to read these to gain a greater understanding of EBP.

Essentially, there are four stages to the EBP process (Flemming, 2008) which are relevant no matter which area of nursing you are working in:

1. Clinical uncertainty from practice is turned into a focused question.

2. The components of the focused question are used as a basis for literature searching to identify relevant research evidence.

3. The identified research evidence is appraised to assess its methodological quality and limitations.

4. The best available evidence is considered alongside your clinical expertise, the preferences of the patient and, where applicable, the available resources.

Let's look at each of these stages in turn.

1. Clinical uncertainty from practice is turned into a focused question

In trying to find some research, the first thing you need to establish is what the question is that you are trying to answer. This is different to identifying a research question that would lead to you undertaking the research yourself. This type of question development is about focusing the question you want to ask prior to starting any searching in computer databases or the library. What you want to do by focusing your question is to transfer this, through searching, into high-quality, relevant research and avoiding wading through hundreds of irrelevant papers. Developing a focused question for literature searching can save a great deal of searching time.

There are a number of different question formulation frameworks that can help you focus your question; which one you use depends on the kind of question you are asking. If you are interested in 'what works'-type questions – that is, questions about the effectiveness of interventions, best answered by a randomised controlled trial or a systematic review of randomised controlled trials – then the format of the PICO framework will work well for you (Straus et al., 2018). PICO stands for:

P – patient or population

I – intervention

C – counter-intervention (where relevant, if not leave out)

O – outcome.

Relating this framework to Stephan's situation, we know that he is experiencing troubling pain as a result of his advanced bone cancer. We may be interested in knowing if Stephan used a pain diary to regularly record the severity of his pain, whether this may help both his ability to report his pain and subsequently its treatment. In this case, using the PICO framework to focus this question would be helpful:

P – people with pain from advanced bone cancer

I – using a pain diary to record the severity of pain

C – not using a pain diary

O – improved pain control achieved by better reporting.

This leads to the focused question: 'Do people experiencing pain from advanced bone cancer who record the severity of their pain in a pain diary have improved pain control?'

PICO is less well suited, however, if we are interested in questions about people's experiences of healthcare, a particular illness, or situation. For these kinds of questions the question formulation framework SPICE can be helpful (Booth, 2006). SPICE, which is more appropriate for use with qualitative research, stands for:

S – setting

P – perspective

I – interest, phenomenon of

C – comparison

E – evaluation.

If we think about Stephan's direct question above, he wishes to know more about other people's experiences of taking part in research studies. He is also interested in knowing about the experiences of people's near relatives. This is a very suitable question to use the SPICE framework for:

S – home, hospice, hospital setting

P – people with a life-limiting condition nearing the end of their life and/or those close to them

I – participation in research study

C – (by implication only) not taking part in research – this does not always need completing

E – individual's experiences, benefits, disadvantages.

Using the SPICE framework leads to the focused question: 'What are the benefits and disadvantages of taking part in research studies for people with life-limiting conditions and who are nearing the end of their lives?'

Thinking of Stephan's wish to understand more about the impact of him taking part in research on his partner Michael, the question could be rephrased: 'What are the experiences of relatives of people with life-limiting conditions who chose to participate in research near the end of their lives?'

Developing a focused question provides you with the key terms and concepts that can be used within your literature searching. Practice applying this technique in Activity 8.4.

Activity 8.4 Critical thinking

Think about an aspect of clinical practice relating to people with life-limiting conditions or at the end of life where you weren't sure of an answer to a patient's question, why a procedure was undertaken in a particular way, or why a particular treatment or intervention was being given to a patient etc. (a clinical uncertainty). Try to frame this uncertainty into a focused question using either the PICO or SPICE frameworks.

There is no answer provided as this exercise is based on your own example.

Activity 8.4 encouraged you to develop a focused question from clinical uncertainty as the first step in the evidence-based practice process. We now turn to step 2.

2. The components of the focused question are used as a basis for literature searching to identify relevant research evidence

Searching for evidence, particularly that which is high quality, can be time consuming. Having a sense of what you are looking for before starting to search is a bit like writing a shopping list before you go shopping: it enables you to think through what you are looking for before you start, can help keep you focused and stop you getting distracted or looking in the wrong place!

The key words/terms or concepts identified through developing your focused question form the basis of your searching 'shopping list'. You will need to think about where you want to search to find the research literature you are interested in. Most university libraries subscribe to a series of health-related electronic databases which may well contain the kind of research that you are looking for. In general, the key databases include:

CINAHL: Cumulative Index of Nursing and Allied Health Literature – considered to be one of the most relevant databases for nurses and allied health professionals and contains records from 1982 onwards. It indexes the majority of nursing journals and, while it is smaller than MEDLINE, may contain resources that are more relevant to nursing (McKibbon and Marks, 2008).

MEDLINE: Medical Literature Analysis and Retrieval System Online – is the largest international healthcare database. It is produced by the United States National Library of Medicine. It contains records from 1966 and indexes a vast array of medical and other healthcare journals, including nursing journals (McKibbon and Marks, 2008).

Cochrane Library: The Cochrane Library is a series of databases that contains high-quality, independent research evidence. The databases within the Cochrane Library contain different types of research evidence. The one that may be of most use to you is the *Cochrane Database of Systematic Reviews* which is the leading international repository of systematic reviews for healthcare and includes many reviews relevant to nursing.

Your university library will also have electronic access to many hundreds of health-related journals, databases, websites and other sources of information. Asking your subject librarian for information about the resources available to you can be a really good way to start your searching.

The terms and concepts that feature in your focused question form the basis of the key words and phrases you will use when searching within the databases. The methods for searching within each of the databases can vary, but the general principles are the same: use your key words and see if they can be combined in any way. The Boolean operators AND, OR and NOT will also help you to undertake efficient searching.

Thinking back to Stephan's situation we can use the focused question: 'Do people experiencing pain from advanced bone cancer who record the severity of their pain in a pain diary have improved pain control?' to pick out some key words to combine in our search.

If we search for the term 'pain' in one of the major databases, such as CINAHL, then it will return many tens of thousands of results. But we can narrow it down by combining it with another term using the word 'AND'. For example, 'pain' AND 'advanced cancer' will search for sources that use both key words enabling you to identify information that is more relevant to your question.

Using the term 'OR' enables you to broaden your search and look for two similar ways of phrasing the same concept. In our example we might be interested in looking for 'pain diary' OR 'pain chart', which will ensure both pain diaries and pain charts will be included in your search results. This broadens your search results.

Finally, using the term 'NOT' excludes key words that you don't want, and therefore is another way of narrowing your search. You should use it cautiously as it may remove results that might be of interest.

What is key to any successful searching attempt is to plan what you want to look for (i.e., develop a focused question), be systematic in your approach (use key terms and combine them appropriately) and to know where to look to best find the evidence you are seeking to answer your question (which databases are best for the question you have). Searching isn't an exact science, but by using a considered and systematic approach you are more likely to find sources of evidence that are relevant to your question.

Activity 8.5   Evidence-based practice and research

Use the focused question you developed in Activity 8.4 and select a research database to search. Undertake a search using the Boolean operators to narrow, or broaden your search as needed. Don't be put off if you are not successful the first time as developing searching skills takes practice. It may be that you need to try different ways of using your search terms or Boolean operators. From your final results select one paper and read this.

There are no answers provided to this activity, as it is based on your own search.

In Activity 8.5 you have identified a research paper. You can now move to the next step, which is to evaluate the quality of this.

3. The identified research evidence is appraised to assess its methodological quality and limitations

Once you have identified some key papers from your searching that you think may help answer your question, it is important to assess them to determine how well the research was conducted. Before applying the findings from any piece of research into your practice, you need to assess whether the research was conducted in a way that means that the results are valid, reliable and applicable (Ellis, 2019).

By **valid** we mean that any tool used to collect data measures what it is supposed to measure.

By **reliable** we mean when a data collection tool is used repeatedly it produces broadly similar results when used in a similar way, with a similar population. This is particularly relevant in quantitative research.

By **applicable** we mean how well the findings from a particular piece of research can be applied more broadly to others in a similar position or population.

There are a number of approaches to appraising the quality of research, but one approach developed specifically to support clinicians assessing the quality of research is that of the checklists produced by the Critical Appraisal Skills Programme (CASP). These are freely available and can support you in systematically assessing the trustworthiness, relevance and results of published research papers. In Activity 8.6 you will look at the CASP checklists.

Activity 8.6 Evidence-based practice and research

Go to the CASP website (listed at the end of the chapter) and identify the different research methodologies that are covered by the checklists. Choose the checklist that relates to the methodology of the research paper you have read in Activity 8.5 and go through this to see how the structure of the questions asked enables you to consider each component of the paper and start to consider the quality of the paper that you found.

There is no answer provided to this question as this activity is based on your own application of the CASP tools.

Activity 8.6 encouraged you to apply the CASP tools to the paper that you have read. The CASP tools are useful in considering in some depth the methodological quality (i.e., whether it is 'sound') of the research papers that you read. They do require underpinning knowledge of the different research paradigms and research methods to apply these tools effectively, so it is important to continue to develop your knowledge of these things.

4. The best available evidence is considered alongside your clinical expertise, the preferences of the patient and, where applicable, the available resources

If, once you have appraised the piece of research you have identified, you are confident that it is methodologically sound, you can then look to use the findings to inform your practice. In Activity 8.6 you will have seen that some of the questions within the CASP checklists will have led you to consider some key issues – for example, 'Will results will help locally?' and whether the people who were part of the research study are similar enough to the people you are looking after for the results to be applicable. Some of the CASP checklists also ask you to consider what resources (if any) might be needed to implement any change recommended by the research.

Therefore, the final stage of the EBP process is to consider the research evidence you have found in light of these broader questions. EBP is not simply about the research evidence 'telling you what to do', but it is about using research evidence as one source of information for decision-making and underpinning practice. When thinking about using research evidence to help inform your practice, using the evidence-based practice 'jigsaw' can help you consider the place of research in supporting clinical decisions. You can see this in Figure 8.1.

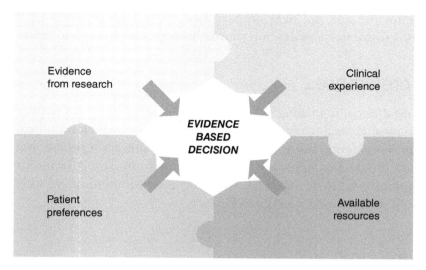

Figure 8.1 Evidence-based practice 'jigsaw'

Source: Adapted from Cullum et al., 2007.

In the 'jigsaw' you can see how evidence from research is one component of an evidence-based decision. Let's briefly look at the others.

Clinical experience and expertise

Your clinical experience and expertise are key to an evidence-based decision. This part of the EBP jigsaw is sometimes misunderstood to mean that the nurse's expertise can overrule what research says, and therefore that an experienced nurse can ignore the research evidence and do what they think best. This is not the case and would be an example of not practising to the NMC standards. Rather, the nurse uses their clinical experience and expertise in a range of other ways such as:

- communicating effectively with the patient to support them in exploring how the evidence applies to their circumstances, wishes and preferences;
- undertaking holistic patient assessment and using evidence to support person-centred care planning;
- identifying uncertainty which requires review of the evidence base;
- collaborating with the interdisciplinary team to develop treatment and care plans and to improve the service;
- maintaining their skills of EBP.

As a student, you are developing your skills in all of these areas and will continue to develop these throughout your career. You may feel you have little to contribute currently in terms of your clinical experience and expertise; this isn't the case. By speaking to your patients and getting to know them and their concerns, you can start to understand what is important to them and how your professional knowledge and skills, however junior you are, can help support them. Your skills in accessing the evidence base will also ensure that you develop your knowledge based on good information.

Patient preferences

Patient-focused decision-making is key to person-centred care and patient preference is central to most clinical decisions. Sometimes, evidence may indicate that a particular treatment or intervention will lead to the better outcomes for a patient, but the patient may not want to take that approach in their treatment or care. Where this is the case, different options need to be explored, alongside good communication with the patient, to understand their concerns and goals for care.

Research summary: people's participation in research at the end of life

Vickova, K, Polakova, K, Tuckova, A, Houska, A and Loucka, M (2021) Views of patients with advanced disease and their relatives on participation in palliative care research. *BMC Palliative Care*, 20(1): 1–7.

What?

To explore how patients with advanced disease and their relatives evaluate their experience of research participation.

How?

Data from a survey including open-ended questions of 170 people with advanced disease and 108 relatives in hospital in the Czech Republic and a longitudinal cohort study.

What did they find?

48 per cent of people 'didn't mind' taking part in research.

51 per cent of people found it interesting.

Additionally, motivation for participation was influenced by: an individual's wish to improve care for other patients, realising it may not help them; to support research endeavours so knowledge could be developed in the field; to express their own opinions about care. It was also found that when patients and their families trusted the researchers or the staff asking them to take part, they were keener to participate.

The research summarised above will help to answer the uncertainty posed by Stephan's question. Activity 8.7 encourages you to apply this to Stephan's situation.

Activity 8.7   Reflection

Think back to Stephan's situation. He posed a question as to how other people at the end of life have found the experience of taking part in research. He also wondered what it might be like for his partner Michael.

Using the detail of the research provided in the research summary above, think how you might be able to use these findings to help support Stephan in his decision-making about taking part in the research study.

There are no answers provided to this question as it is based on your own application of the evidence.

Chapter summary

In this chapter we have begun to explore the importance of evidence-based practice and the role of research in palliative and end of life care and have considered how this evidence base might be developed and used. We have placed the patient at the centre of all research and focused on the significance of their contributions to research studies when they are nearing the end of their life.

We have explored types of research that can be used to answer different clinical uncertainties and research questions and looked at how research questions may be generated from clinical practice.

Finally, we have explored how you can find, appraise and apply research in your clinical practice, using the evidence-based practice process. This process underpins your clinical decision-making and central to this is the importance of including the patient and those important to them in all elements of their care.

Activities: brief outline answers

Activity 8.2   Evidence-based practice and research (page 143)

Question 1 is best answered by quantitative research that tests which forms of analgesia are most effective for bone pain.

Question 2 is best answered by qualitative research that explores the views and experiences of people who have life-limiting illness in relation to taking part in research.

Activity 8.3   Evidence-based practice and research (page 144)

This is a reflective activity and based on your own views, so no definitive answer is provided. Some things to consider in response to Stephan's question include speaking with a research nurse in the clinical setting you are working in (if one is available) or searching for some research literature which explores people's experiences of taking part in research.

Further reading

These texts explore EBN and research in detail:

Ellis, P (2022a) Critiquing research: approach-specific elements, in Ellis, P (2022) *Evidence-based Practice in Nursing* (5th edn). London: Sage, 65–86.

Ellis, P (2022b) *Evidence-based Practice in Nursing* (5th edn). London: Sage.

Aveyard, H and Sharpe, H (2017) *A Beginner's Guide to Evidence-Based Practice in Health and Social Care.* London: McGraw Hill Education.

Useful websites

casp-uk.net/

The Critical Appraisal Skills Programme (CASP) includes critical skills appraisal tools, or checklists for different types of research methodologies, which are useful tools to support your critical appraisal of research.

uk.cochrane.org/evidence-nursing

Launched in 2015, this is an ongoing series of evidence and other resources that relate to nursing practice.

ebn.bmj.com

The home of the journal *Evidence-based Nursing* which publishes critical commentaries and summaries of a range of research that relates to nursing practice.

Glossary

Aetiology: The causes of a disease.

Assisted suicide: The act of deliberately assisting another person to kill themselves.

Autonomy: The right to make decisions about your own life.

Compassionate engagement: Engaging with someone in a sensitive and holistic way that recognises their suffering and with a willingness to improve their situation, and creating opportunity for them to find purpose and meaning in life.

Cultural competence: Being sensitive to people's cultural heritage and identity, and being responsive to beliefs and conventions that are aligned with this (Care Quality Commission, 2022).

Curative care: Curative care includes treatments that may potentially cure or modify the disease. This can run alongside palliative care.

Delirium: A physiological consequence of disease or treatments which presents as disturbed consciousness, inattention and cognitive impairment.

Distress: A state of suffering caused by physical or emotional pain.

Emotional intelligence: Being able to recognise and respond to emotions in self and others.

Equitable: Being fair. This is different from equality, which means treating everyone the same.

End of life care: End of life care is part of palliative care and is for people who are in the final weeks, days or hours of life. End of life care aims to help people live as comfortably as possible, by managing physical symptoms and providing emotional support.

Euthanasia: The act of deliberately ending a person's life to relieve their suffering.

Holistic: Considering the person as a 'whole', as opposed to considering issues or problems in isolation – for example, giving someone a medication for a symptom and also considering psychosocial-spiritual issues which may be contributing to that symptom.

Hospice: Hospice care specialises in care of people who have advanced life-limiting conditions and their families. Care is provided in a range of locations including the hospice, people's home, care homes and through outreach services. The majority of hospices in the UK are charities, many of which receive some NHS funding.

Integrated care systems: Where different providers of health and social care work together to enable continuity and coordination of care. The aim of this is to improve patient experience, efficiency and value in healthcare delivery systems (Health Foundation, 2016).

Life-limiting illness: An incurable condition/illness which will shorten a person's life.

Multimorbidity: Where someone has two or more long-term conditions.

Palliative care: An approach to care for people with life-limiting illness and at the end of life and their families and carers that aims to relieve distress and promote quality of life.

Person-centred care: Working in partnership with the person to plan and deliver care that aligns with their goals, wishes, values and preferences.

Personalised care: An approach to care that aims to give people more control over their health and more personalised care. Discussed as part of the NHS Long Term Plan (2019).

Progressive illness: Progressive illnesses will get worse over time. The pace of health decline will vary on the type of illness experienced.

Resilience: Being able to adapt to change and cope with difficulties or setbacks.

Specialist palliative care: Palliative care provided by people who specialise in this type of care. Often required for more complex problems.

Spirituality: Has different meanings to different people. It involves having connections with things beyond the self that contribute to life's meaning and can contribute to feelings of peace. For some spiritual life relates to religion, for others it may involve mindful connections with other things such as nature or community.

Wellbeing: A subjective experience that is influenced by physical and mental health, feelings of self-worth, spirituality, the environments life is lived in, relationships, dignity, emotions and meaning in life.

References

Academy of Medical Sciences and Ipsos MORI (2019) *The Departure Lounge: Public Attitudes to Death and Dying*. Available online at: www.ipsos.com/en-uk/departure-lounge-public-attitudes-death-and-dying (accessed 21 October 2022).

Anandarajah, G and Hight, E (2001) Spirituality and medical practice: using the HOPE questions as a practical tool for spiritual assessment. *American Family Physician*, 63(1): 81–89.

Alzheimer's Society (2021) *Dementia, Advance Decisions and Advance Statements*. Available online at: www.alzheimers.org.uk/get-support/legal-financial/dementia-advance-decisions-statements (accessed 21 October 2022).

Bajwah, S, Koffman, J, Hussain, J, Bradshaw, A, Hocaoglu, M et al. (2021) Specialist palliative care services response to ethnic minority groups with Covid-19: equal but inequitable – an observational study. *BMJ Supportive and Palliative Care*. Published online: 12 September 2021. doi: 10.1136/bmjspcare-2021-003083

BBC (2018) *Dying is Not as Bad as You Think*. Available online at: www.bbc.co.uk/ideas/videos/dying-is-not-as-bad-as-you-think/p062m0xt (accessed 21 October 2022).

Booth, A (2006) Clear and present questions: formulating questions for evidence based practice. *Library Hi Tech*, 24(3): 355–368.

Cain, C, Surbone, A, Elk, R and Kagawa-Singer, M (2018) Culture and palliative care: preferences, communication, meaning, and mutual decision making. *Journal of Pain and Symptom Management*, 55(5):1408–1419.

Carduff, E, Johnston, S, Winstanley, C, Morrish, J, Murray, S et al. (2018) What does 'complex' mean in palliative care? Triangulating qualitative findings from 3 settings. *BMC Palliative Care*, 17(12): 1–7.

Care Quality Commission (2022) Culturally appropriate care. Available online at: www.cqc.org.uk/guidance-providers/adult-social-care/culturally-appropriate-care (accessed 21 October 2022).

Caswell, G and O'Connor, M (2019) 'I've no fear of dying alone': exploring perspectives on living and dying alone. *Mortality*, 24(1): 17–31.

Cedar, D and Walker, G (2020) Protecting the wellbeing of nurses providing end-of-life care. *Nursing Times*,116(2): 36–40.

Choudry, M, Latif, A and Warburton, K (2018) An overview of the spiritual importance of end-of-life care among the five major faiths of the United Kingdom. *Clinical Medicine*, 18(1): 23–31.

Clark, D (2010) International progress in creating palliative medicine as a specialized discipline, in Hanks, G, Cherny, N, Christakis, N, Fallon, M, Kaasa, S and Pertenoy, R (eds), *Oxford Textbook of Palliative Medicine* (4th edn). Oxford: Oxford University Press, 9–16.

Cochrane Library (2022) *The Cochrane Library.* Available online at: www.cochranelibrary.com/ (accessed 21 October 2022).

Critical Appraisal Skills Programme (2022) *CASP Checklists.* Available online at: www.casp-uk.net/casp-tools-checklists/ (accessed 21 October 2022).

Cruise (2022) *Complicated Grief.* Available online at: www.cruse.org.uk/understanding-grief/effects-of-grief/complicated-grief/ (accessed 21 October 2022).

Cullum N, DiCenso A, and Ciliska, D (2007) *Evidence-based Nursing: An Introduction.* London: Wiley-Blackwell.

den Herder-van der Eerden, M, Hasselaar, J, Payne, S, Varey, S, Schwabe, S et al. (2017) How continuity of care is experienced within the context of integrated palliative care: a qualitative study with patients and family caregivers in five European countries. *Palliative Medicine,* 31(10): 946–955.

Department of Health (2008) *End of Life Care Strategy: Promoting High Quality Care for All Adults at the End of Life.* Available online at: www.assets.publishing.service.gov.uk/government/uploads/system/uploads/attachment_data/file/136431/End_of_life_strategy.pdf (accessed 21 October 2022).

Ellis, P (2019) Critiquing research: approach-specific elements, in Ellis, P and Standing, M (eds), *Evidence-based Practice in Nursing* (4th edn) London: Sage, 63–84.

Ellis, P and Standing, M (2019) *Evidence-based Practice in Nursing* (4th edn). London: Sage.

Emich, C (2018) Conceptualizing collaboration in nursing. *Nursing Forum,* 53(4): 567–573.

End of Life Think Tank (2021) What matters conversations. Available online at: www.whatmattersconversations.org/ (accessed 21 October 2022).

Fang, C and Tanaka, M (2022) An exploration of person-centred approach in end-of-life care policies in England and Japan. *BMC Palliative Care,* 21(1). doi: 10.1186/s12904-022-00965-w

Fettes, L, Ashford, S and Maddocks, M (2018) *Setting and Implementing Patient-Set Goals in Palliative Care.* King's College London. Available online at: www.kcl.ac.uk/nmpc/assets/rehab/gas-booklet-2018-final.pdf (accessed 21 October 2022).

Finucane, A, Swenson, C, MacArtney, J, Perry, R, Lamberton, H et al. (2021) What makes palliative care needs 'complex'? A multisite sequential explanatory mixed methods study of patients referred for specialist palliative care. *BMC Palliative Care,* 20(1): 18.

Flemming, K (2008) Asking answerable questions, in Cullum, N, Ciliska, D, Haynes, R and Marks, S (eds), *Evidence-based Nursing: An Introduction.* Oxford: Blackwell, 18–23.

Flemming, K, Atkin, K, Ward, C and Watt, I (2019) Adult family carers' perceptions of their educational needs when providing end-of-life care: a systematic review of qualitative research. *AMRC Open Research,* 1(2):1–26.

Ford, C (2019) Adult pain assessment and management. *British Journal of Nursing*, 28(7). doi: 10.12968/bjon.2019.28.7.421

Fraser, S and Greenhalgh, T (2001) Coping with complexity: educating for capability. *British Medical Journal*, 323(7316): 799–803.

Frimley Health and Care (2021) *A Guide to Reaching our Communities in End of Life Care.* Available online at: www.eastberkshireccg.nhs.uk/doclink/frimley-community-end-of-life-booklet/eyJ0eXAiOiJKV1QiLCJhbGciOiJIUzI1NiJ9.eyJzdWIiOiJmcmlttbGV5LWNvbW11bml0eS1lbmQtb2YtGlmZS1ib29rbGV0IiwiaWF0IjoxNjM2OTTkxNTczLCJleHAiOjE2MzcwNzc5NzN9.G2Ppp2KEPNIUndYyXLvg4P0lacC3i_m5hec5uj1qkG8 (accessed 21 October 2022).

Fringer, A, Hechinger, M and Schnepp, W (2018) Transitions as experienced by persons in palliative care circumstances and their families: a qualitative meta-synthesis. *BMC Palliative Care*, 17(1). doi:10.1186/s12904-018-0275-7

Gerber, K, Hayes, B and Bryant, C (2019) 'It all depends!': a qualitative study of preferences for place of care and place of death in terminally ill patients and their family caregivers. *Palliative Medicine*, 33(7): 802–811.

Givler, A, Bhatt, H and Maani-Fogelman, A (2021) *The Importance of Cultural Competence in Pain and Palliative Care.* Treasure Island, FL: StatPearls.

Goodrich, J and Cornwell, J (2008) *Seeing the Person in the Patient. The Point of Care Review Paper.* London: Kings Fund.

gov.uk (2014) The Health and Social Care Act 2008 (Regulated Activities) Regulations 2014. Available online at: www.legislation.gov.uk/ukdsi/2014/9780111117613/contents (accessed 21 October 2022).

Hanks, S, Neve, H and Gale, T (2021) Preparing health profession students for practice in complex real world settings: how do educators respond to a model of capability? *International Journal of Practice-based Learning in Health and Social Care*, 9(1): 50–63.

Harding, E, Wait, S and Scrutton, J (2015) *The State of Play in Person-centred Care.* Health Policy Partnership. Available online at: www.healthpolicypartnership.com/app/uploads/The-state-of-play-in-person-centred-care-summary.pdf (accessed 21 October 2022).

Hardoon, D, Hey, N and Brunetti, S (2020) *Wellbeing Evidence at the Heart of Policy.* What Works Wellbeing. Available online at: www.whatworkswellbeing.org/resources/wellbeing-evidence-at-the-heart-of-policy/ (accessed 21 October 2022).

Hardy, B (2018) Meeting the needs of carers of people at the end of life. *Nursing Standard*, 33(1): 59–66.

Hardy, B, King, N and Rodriguez, A (2014) The experiences of patients and carers in the daily management of care at the end of life. *International Journal of Palliative Nursing*, 20(12): 591–598.

Harris, J, Booth, A, Cargo, M, Hannes, K, Harden, A et al. (2018) Cochrane Qualitative and Implementation Methods Group guidance series – paper 2: methods for question formulation, searching and protocol development for qualitative evidence synthesis. *Journal of Clinical Epidemiology*, 97: 39–48.

Hawthorne, D and Yurkovich, N (2003) Human relationship: the forgotten dynamic in palliative care. *Palliative and Supportive Care,* 1(3): 261–265.

Health Foundation (2016) *Person-centred Care Made Simple: What Everyone Should Know about Person-centred Care.* London: Health Foundation. Available online at: www.health. org.uk/publications/person-centred-care-made-simple (accessed 1 December 2022).

Heffernan, M, Quinn Griffin, M, McNulty, R and Fitzpatrick, J (2010) Self-compassion and emotional intelligence in nurses. *International Journal of Nursing Practice,* 16(4): 366–73.

Higginson, I (2016) Research challenges in palliative and end of life care. *BMJ Supportive and Palliative Care,* 6: 2–4.

Hockley, J (2008) Personhood and identity in palliative care, in Payne, S, Seymour, J and Ingleton, C (eds), *Palliative Care Principles and Evidence for Practice* (2nd edn). London: Open University Press McGraw-Hill Education, 347–361.

Hopkins, S, Lovick, R, Polak, L, Bowers, B, Morgan, T, Kelly, P and Barclay, S (2020) Reassessing advance care planning in the light of Covid-19. *British Medical Journal,* 369. doi:10.1136/bmj.m1927

Hospice UK (2021) *Equality in Hospice and End of Life Care: Challenges and Change.* London: Hospice UK.

Hospice UK (2022) *Care After Death* (4th edn). London: Hospice UK.

Hussain, J, Koffman, J and Bajwah, S (2021) Racism and palliative care. *Palliative Medicine,* 35(5): 810–813.

Inbadas, H (2018) Spirituality, spiritual care and the role of nurses in palliative care, in Walshe, C, Preston, N and Johnston, B (eds), *Palliative Care Nursing, Principles and Evidence for Practice* (3rd edn). London: Open University Press McGraw-Hill Education.

James, R, Flemming, K, Hodson, M and Oxlet, T (2021) Palliative care for homeless and vulnerably housed people: scoping review and thematic analysis. *BMJ Supportive and Palliative Care.* Published online, doi: 10.1136/bmjspcare-2021-003020

James Lind Alliance (2021) Palliative and end of life care Priority Setting Partnership (PeolcPSP). www.jla.nihr.ac.uk/priority-setting-partnerships/palliative-and-end-of-life-care/ (James Lind Alliance (2022) accessed 25 November 2022).

About us. Available online at: www.jla.nihr.ac.uk/about-the-james-lind-alliance (accessed 21 October 2022).

Kennedy, C, Brooks-Young, P, Gray, C, Larkin, P, Connolly, M et al. (2014) Diagnosing dying: an integrative literature review. *BMJ Supportive and Palliative Care,* 4: 263–270.

Kennedy, P, Hudson, B, Shulman, C. and Brophy, N (2018) *A Toolkit for Supporting Homeless People with Advanced Ill Health.* Available online at: www.homelesspalliativecare. com (accessed 21 October 2022).

King, N, Bravington, A, Brooks, J, Hardy, B, Melvin, J et al. (2013) The Pictor technique: a method for exploring the experience of collaborative working. *Qualitative Health Research,* 23(8): 1138–1152.

Kingdon, A, Spathis, A, Brodrick, R, Clarke, G, Kuhn, I et al. (2021) What is the impact of clinically assisted hydration in the last days of life? A systematic literature review and narrative synthesis. *BMJ Supportive and Palliative Care*, 11: 68–74.

Krishna, L and Kwek, S (2015) The changing face of personhood at the end of life: the ring theory of personhood. *Palliative and Supportive Care*, 13(4): 1123–1129.

Leadership Alliance for the Care of Dying People (2014) *One Chance to Get it Right: Improving People's Experience of Care in the Last Few Days and Hours of Life.* Available online at: www.assets.publishing.service.gov.uk/government/uploads/system/uploads/attachment_data/file/323188/One_chance_to_get_it_right.pdf (accessed 21 October 2022).

Lichtner, V, Dowding, D, Esterhuizen, P, Closs, J, Long, A et al. (2014) Pain assessment for people with dementia: a systematic review of systemic reviews of pain assessment tools. *BMC Geriatrics*, 14: 138.

Lynn, J and Adamson, D (2003) *Living Well at the End of Life: Adapting Health Care to Serious Chronic Illness in Old Age.* Santa Monica: Rand Health.

Lyons, H (2021) P-5 Improving palliative and end-of-life support for those who are homeless and vulnerably housed. *BMJ Supportive and Palliative Care*, 11: A11.

Manning, E and Gagnon, M (2017) The complex patient: a concept clarification. *Nursing and Health Sciences*, 19(1): 13–21.

Mannix, K (2018) *With the End in Mind: How to Live and Die Well.* London: HarperCollins.

Mannix, K (2021) *Listen: How to Find the Words for Tender Conversations.* London: HarperCollins.

Marie Curie (2022a) *Continence Care in Palliative Care.* Available online at: www.mariecurie.org.uk/professionals/palliative-care-knowledge-zone/symptom-control/continence-care#:~:text=In%20the%20last%20few%20hours,may%20feel%20agitated%20and%20restless (accessed 21 October 2022).

Marie Curie (2022b) *Palliative and End of Life Care Needs for People with Learning Disabilities.* Available online at: www.mariecurie.org.uk/professionals/palliative-care-knowledge-zone/proving-good-quality-care/learning-disability (accessed 21 October 2022).

Marie Curie (2022c) *Providing Spiritual Care.* Available online at: www.mariecurie.org.uk/professionals/palliative-care-knowledge-zone/individual-needs/spiritual-care?gclid=Cj0KCQiAm5ycBhCXARIsAPldzoWMxcY0yXQyamACRQEQgOwtXiP1F3KTVEEAlEDmh7UZXmRmh1Jk-l0aAjXdEALw_wcB (accessed 30 November 2022).

Mayland, C, Mitchell, S, Flemming, K, Tatnell, L, Roberts, L et al. (2022) Addressing inequitable access to hospice care. *BMJ Supportive and Palliative Care*, 12: 302–304.

McKibbon, K and Marks, S (2008) Searching for the best evidence part 2: Searching CINAHL and MEDLINE, in Cullum, N, Ciliska, D, Haynes, R and Marks, S (eds), *Evidence-based Nursing: An Introduction.* Oxford: Blackwell, 37–47.

Mencap (2022) *What is a Learning Disability.* Available online at: www.mencap.org.uk/learning-disability-explained/what-learning-disability (accessed 21 October 2022).

MIND (2022) *Bereavement.* Available online at: www.mind.org.uk/information-support/guides-to-support-and-services/bereavement/about-bereavement/ (accessed 21 October 2022).

Mitchell, G and Agnelli, J (2015) Person-centred care for people with dementia: Kitwood reconsidered. *Nursing Standard*, 30(7): 46–50.

Mitchell, W (2018) *Somebody I Used to Know.* London: Bloomsbury.

Mochamat, M, Cuhls, H, Sellin, J, Conrad, R, Radbruch, L et al (2021) Fatigue in advanced disease associated with palliative care: A systematic review of non-pharmacological treatments. *Palliative Medicine*, 35(4): 697–709.

Morley, C and Cathala, X (2019) How to appraise qualitative research. *Evidence Based Nursing*, 22(1), doi: 10.1136/ebnurs-2018-103044

Mücke, M, Mochamat, M, Cuhls, H, Peuckmann-Post, V, Minton, O et al. (2015) Pharmacological treatments for fatigue associated with palliative care. *Cochrane Database of Systematic Review*, 5, doi: 10.1002/14651858.CD006788.pub3

Murray, S, Kendall, M, Boyd, K and Sheikh, A (2005) Illness trajectories and palliative care. *British Medical Journal*, 330 (7498): 1007–1011.

National Cancer Research Institute (2015) New Report Highlights Low Levels of Palliative and End of Life Care Research Funding in the UK. Available online at: www.ncri.org.uk/new-report-highlights-low-levels-of-palliative-and-of-life-care-research-funding-in-the-uk/ (accessed 21 October 2022).

National Palliative and End of Life Care Partnership (2021) *Ambitions for Palliative and End of Life Care: A National Framework for Local Action 2021–2026.* Available online at: www.endoflifeambitions.co.uk (accessed 21 October 2022).

National Institute for Health Research (NIHR) (2017) *Comprehensive Care: Older People Living with Frailty in Hospitals.* Available online at: www.evidence.nihr.ac.uk/themedreview/comprehensive-care-older-people-with-frailty-in-hospital/ (accessed 21 October 2022).

Nelson, A (2011) What is a randomised controlled trial? *Evidence-based Nursing*, 14(4): 97–8.

NHS (2019) The NHS Long Term Plan. Available online at: www.longtermplan.nhs.uk/publication/nhs-long-term-plan/ (accessed 21 October 2022).

NHS (2021) Mental Capacity Act. Available online at: www.nhs.uk/conditions/social-care-and-support-guide/making-decisions-for-someone-else/mental-capacity-act/ (accessed 21 October 2022).

NHS Digital (2019) *Health and Care of People with Learning Disabilities.* Available online at: www.digital.nhs.uk/data-and-information/publications/statistical/health-and-care-of-people-with-learning-disabilities (accessed 21 October 2022).

NHS England (2015) *NHS Chaplaincy Guidelines 2015: Promoting Excellence in Pastoral, Spiritual and Religious Care.* Available online at: www.england.nhs.uk/wp-content/uploads/2015/03/nhs-chaplaincy-guidelines-2015.pdf (accessed 21 October 2022).

NHS England (2016) *NHS England Specialist Level Palliative Care: Information for Commissioners.* Available online at: www.england.nhs.uk/wp-content/uploads/2016/04/speclst-palliatv-care-comms-guid.pdf (accessed 21 October 2022).

NHS England (2017) *Delivering High Quality End of Life Care for People Who Have a Learning Disability: Resources and Tips for Commissioners, Service Providers and Health and Social Care Staff.* Available online at: www.england.nhs.uk/wp-content/uploads/2017/08/delivering-end-of-life-care-for-people-with-learning-disability.pdf (accessed 21 October 2022).

NHS England (2022) *Who is Considered a Carer?* Available online at: www.england.nhs.uk/commissioning/comm-carers/carers/ (accessed 21 October 2022).

NHS Scotland (2009) *Spiritual Care Matters: An Introductory Resource for All NHS Scotland Staff.* Edinburgh: NHS Education for Scotland.

NHS Scotland (2020) *Scottish Palliative Care Guidelines: Delirium.* Available online at: www.palliativecareguidelines.scot.nhs.uk/guidelines/symptom-control/Delirium.aspx (accessed 30 November 2022).

NICE (2015) *Care of Dying Adults in the Last Days of Life.* Available online at: www.nice.org.uk/guidance/ng31 (accessed 21 October 2022).

NICE (2018) *Clinical Knowledge Summaries. Cardiac Arrest: Out of Hospital Care.* Available online at: cks.nice.org.uk/topics/cardiac-arrest-out-of-hospital-care/ (accessed 21 October 2022).

NICE (2019) *Delirium: Prevention, Diagnosis and Management.* Available online at: www.nice.org.uk/guidance/cg103/chapter/Recommendations#risk-factor-assessment-2 (accessed 21 October 2022).

NICE (2021a) *Clinical Knowledge Summaries. Palliative Care: Nausea and Vomiting.* Available online at: cks.nice.org.uk/topics/palliative-care-nausea-vomiting/ (accessed 21 October 2022).

NICE (2021b) *Clinical Knowledge Summaries. Palliative Care: Oral.* Available online at: cks.nice.org.uk/topics/palliative-care-oral/ (accessed 21 October 2022).

NICE (2022) *Clinical Knowledge Summaries. Scenario: Communication.* Available online at: cks.nice.org.uk/topics/palliative-care-general-issues/management/communication/ (accessed 21 October 2022).

NIHR (2022) *End of Life Care: Research Highlights the Importance of Conversations and Need for Equal Access.* Available online at: evidence.nihr.ac.uk/collection/end-of-life-care-research-highlights-the-importance-of-conversations-and-need-for-equal-access/ (accessed 30 November 2022).

NMC (2018) *Future Nurse: Standards of Proficiency for Registered Nurses.* Available online at: www.nmc.org.uk/globalassets/sitedocuments/standards-of-proficiency/nurses/future-nurse-proficiencies.pdf (accessed 23 November 2022).

NMC (2021) *Continuing Professional Development.* Available online at: www.nmc.org.uk/revalidation/requirements/cpd/ (accessed 21 October 2022).

Ntizimira, C, Deo, M, Dunne, M and Krakauer (2022) Decolonizing end-of-life care: lessons and opportunities. *ecancer,* 16: ed121.

Nuffield Trust (2021) *Quality Watch: Cancer Survival Rates.* Available online at: www.nuffieldtrust.org.uk/resource/cancer-survival-rates (accessed 21 October 2022).

O'Donnell, S, Bone, A, Finucane, A, McAleese, J, Higginson, I et al. (2021) Changes in mortality patterns and place of death during the Covid-19 pandemic: a descriptive analysis of mortality data across four nations. *Palliative Medicine*, 35(10): 1975–1984.

Office for National Statistics (ONS) (2019) *The Cost of Living Alone.* Available online at: www.ons.gov.uk/peoplepopulationandcommunity/birthsdeathsandmarriages/families/articles/thecostoflivingalone/2019-04-04#:~:text=More%20and%20more%20of%20us,rise%20to%2010.7%20million2 (accessed 21 October 2022).

Office for National Statistics (ONS) (2020) *Five-year Average Weekly Deaths by Place of Death, England and Wales, Deaths Occurring Between 2015 and 2019.* Available online at: www.ons.gov.uk/peoplepopulationandcommunity/birthsdeathsandmarriages/deaths/adhocs/11622fiveyearaverageweeklydeathsbyplaceofdeathenglandandwalesdeaths-occurringbetween2015and2019 (accessed 21 October 2022).

Office for National Statistics (ONS) (2021) *Deaths Registered in England and Wales 2020.* Available online at: www.ons.gov.uk/peoplepopulationandcommunity/birthsdeaths-andmarriages/deaths/bulletins/deathsregistrationsummarytables/2020 (accessed 21 October 2022).

Öhlén, J, Reimer-Kirkham, S, Astle, B, Hakanson, C, Lee, J et al. (2017) Person-centred care dialectics: inquired in the context of palliative care. *Nursing Philosophy*, 18(4), doi: 10.1111/nup.12177

Oliver, D (2015) *Short Biography of Dame Cicely Saunders.* Available online at: www.cicelysaundersarchive.wordpress.com/tag/david-tasma/ (accessed 21 October 2022).

Oxford English Dictionary (2022) *Oxford English Dictionary.* Available online at: www.OED.com (accessed 21 October 2022).

Pask, S, Pinto, C, Bristow, K, van Vliet, L, Nicholson, C et al. (2018) A framework for complexity in palliative care: a qualitative study with patients, family carers and professionals. *Palliative Medicine*, 32(6): 1078–1090.

Pattison, N, Deaton, C and McCabe, C (2021) Florence Nightingale's legacy for clinical academics: a framework analysis of a clinical professorial network and a model for clinical academia. *Journal of Clinical Nursing*, 31(3–4): 353–361.

Perkins, G, Nolan, J, Soar, J, Hawkes, C, Wyllie, J et al. (2021) *Epidemiology of Cardiac Arrest Guidelines.* Available online at: www.resus.org.uk/library/2021-resuscitation-guidelines/epidemiology-cardiac-arrest-guidelines#:~:text=Post%2Dresuscitation%20care&text=Approximately%20half%20of%20those%20admitted,who%20survive%20are%20discharged%20home (accessed 21 October 2022).

Porter, l, Steel, J, Fairclough, T, LeBlanc,T, Bull, J et al. (2021) Caregiver-guided pain coping skills training for patients with advanced cancer: results from a randomised clinical trial. *Palliative Medicine*, 35(5): 952–961.

Price, B (2019) *Delivering Person-centred Care in Nursing.* London: Sage.

Public Health England (2016) *Faith at the End of Life: A Resource for Professionals, Providers and Commissioners Working in Communities.* London: Public Health England.

QNI (2022) *Introducing Personalised Care.* Available online at: qni.org.uk/nursing-in-the-community/personalised-care/ (accessed 30 November 2022).

Resuscitation Council (2016) *Guidance from the British Medical Association, the Resuscitation Council (UK) and the Royal College of Nursing on Ensuring High-quality Communication, Decision-making and Recording in Relation to Decisions about CPR* (3rd edn). Available online at: www.resus.org.uk/sites/default/files/2020-05/20160123%20Decisions%20Relating%20to%20CPR%20-%202016.pdf (accessed 21 October 2022).

Rietjens, J, Korfage I and Seymour, J (2021) Advance care planning, in Cherny, N, Fallon, M, Kaasa, S, Portenoy, R and Currow, D (eds), *Oxford Textbook of Palliative Medicine* (5th edn). Oxford: Oxford University Press.

Rietjens, J, Sudore, R, Connolly, M, Van Delden, J, Drickamer, M et al. (2017) Definition and recommendations for advance care planning: an international consensus supported by the European Association for Palliative Care. *Lancet Oncology,* 18(9): e543–e551.

Rodríguez-Prat, A, Monforte-Royo, C, Porta-Sales, J, Escribano, X and Balaguer, A (2016) Patient perspectives of dignity, autonomy and control at the end of life: systematic review and meta-ethnography. *PLoS One,* 11(3): e0151435.

Rogers, M and Wattis, J (2015) Spirituality in nursing practice. *Nursing Standard,* 29(39): 51–57.

Rogers, M and Wattis, J (2020) Understanding the role of spirituality in providing person-centred care. *Nursing Standard,* 35(9): 25–30.

Royal College of Nursing (2016) *End of Life Care: Fundamentals of Nursing Care at the End of Life.* Available online at: www.rcn.org.uk/Professional-Development/Professional-services/End-of-life-care-and-wellbeing-for-the-nursing-and-midwifery-workforce (accessed 21 October 2022).

Royal College of Physicians (2021) *End of Life Care in the Acute Care Setting.* London: Royal College of Physicians.

Ryan, T (2022) Facilitators of person and relationship-centred care in nursing. *Nursing Open,* 9(2): 892–899.

Sackett, D, Strauss, S, Richardson, W, Rosenberg, W and Haynes, B (1997) *Evidence Based Medicine: How to Practice and Teach EBM.* Edinburgh: Churchill Livingstone.

Sallnow, L, Smith, R, Ahmedzai, S, Bhadelia, A, Chamerlain, C et al. (2022) Report of the Lancet Commission on the Value of Death: bringing death back into life. *The Lancet,* 399(10327): 837–884.

Sargent, L (2017) Functional Ability, in Giddens, J (ed.), *Concepts for Nursing Practice* (2nd edn). Missouri: Elsevier, 13–20.

Sathiananthan, M, Crawford, G and Eliot, J (2021) Healthcare professionals' perspectives of patient and family preferences of patient place of death: a qualitative study. *BMC Palliative Care,* 20(147), doi: 10.1186/s12904-021-00842-y

Saunders, C (1996) A personal therapeutic journey. *British Medical Journal,* 313(7072): 159–601.

Sekse, R, Hunskår, I and Ellingsen, S (2018) The nurse's role in palliative care: A qualitative meta-synthesis. *Journal of Clinical Nursing*, 27(1–2): e21–38.

Six, S, Bilsen, J and Deschepper, R (2020) Dealing with cultural diversity in palliative care. *BMJ Supportive and Palliative Care*. Published online first, doi: 10.1136/bmjspcare-2020-002511

Skevington, S and Bönke, J (2018) How is subjective well being linked to quality of life? Do we need two concepts and both measures? *Social Science and Medicine*. 206: 21–30.

Soklaridis, S, Ravitz, P, Adler Nevo, G and Lieff, S (2016) Relationship-centred care in health: a 20-year scoping review. *Patient Experience Journal*, 3(10): 130–145.

Steinhauser, K and Tulsky, J (2015) Defining a 'good death', in Cherny, N, Fallon, M, Kaasa, S, Portenoy, R and Currow, D (eds), *Oxford Textbook of Palliative Medicine* (5th edn). Oxford: Oxford University Press.

Straus, S, Glasziou, P, Scott Richardson, W and Haynes, B (2018) *Evidence-based Medicine: How to Practice and Teach EBM* (5th edn). London: Elsevier.

Thomas, J and Harden, A (2008) Methods for the thematic synthesis of qualitative research in systematic reviews. *BMC Medical Research Methodology*, 8(45), doi:10.1186/1471-2288-8-45

Tiberini, R and Richardson, H (2015) *Rehabilitative Palliative Care: Enabling People to Live Fully Until They Die*. London: Hospice UK.

Travers, J, Romero-Ortuno, R, Bailey, J and Cooney, M (2019) Delaying and reversing frailty: a systematic review of primary care interventions. *British Journal of General Practice*, 69(678): e61–e69.

Turner, K and Millington-Sanders, C. on behalf of RCGP and EOLC Partners Think Tank (2022) What Matters Conversations: A 'How to' Guide. Available online at: www.whatmattersconversations.org/a-how-to-guide (accessed 21 October 2022).

Vickova, K, Polakova, K, Tuckova, A, Houska, A and Loucka, M (2021) Views of patients with advanced disease and their relatives on participation in palliative care research. *BMC Palliative Care*, 20(1): 1–7.

Watson, M, Ward, S, Vallath, N, Wells, J, and Campbell, R (2019) *Oxford Handbook of Palliative Care*. Oxford: Oxford University Press.

Wealth Advisor (2020) *Thirty One Million UK Adults Don't Have a Will in Place, Says New Research*. Available online at: www.wealthadviser.co/2020/09/28/290151/thirty-one-million-uk-adults-dont-have-will-place-says-new-research (accessed 21 October 2022).

World Health Organization (WHO) (2018) *Continuity and Coordination of Care: A Practice Brief to Support Implementation of the WHO Framework on Integrated People-centred Health Services*. Available online at: apps.who.int/iris/bitstream/handle/10665/274628/9789241514033-eng.pdf. (accessed 21 October 2022).

World Health Organization (WHO) (2021a) *Quality Health Services and Palliative Care: Practical Approaches and Resources to Support Policy, Strategy and Practice*. Available online at: apps.who.int/iris/bitstream/handle/10665/345674/9789240035164-eng.pdf?sequence=1 (accessed 21 October 2022).

World Health Organization (WHO) (2021b) *Social Determinants of Health*. Available online at: www.who.int/health-topics/social-determinants-of-health#tab=tab_1 (accessed 21 October 2022).

World Health Organization (WHO) (2022) *Palliative Care*. Available online at: www.who.int/news-room/fact-sheets/detail/palliative-care (accessed 21 October 2022).

Index

Academy of Medical Sciences 41–2
activities 4
advance care planning (ACP)
    healthcare professionals 110–11
    MND 116
    overview 109–10
    patients 110
    student nurse responsibilities 114–16
    what matters to you 103–4
advance decisions to refuse treatment (ADRTs) 103,
        108–9, 115
agitation 45
Alzheimer's disease 21
Ambitions for Palliative and End of Life Care 37
Aran case study 41
assisted suicide 116
AtaLoss 55
attentiveness 17
autonomy 26, 29
availability 16

Baha'i faith 34
Bajwah, S 36–7
bereavement and grief 54–5
biological factors 84, 86
blood pressure 45
Boolean operators 148–9
breathing patterns 46
British Medical Association, the Resuscitation
        Council 105

cancer 65, 75
capability 96–7
cardiopulmonary resuscitation (CPR) 103, 104–6
Carduff, E 95
care after death 47
care plans 55–6, 57
carers
    definitions 121–2
    at end of life 130–2
    informal carers 122–4
    information valued by 127–9
    overview 120–1
    supporting 124–7
    what carers say helps them 129–30
Cary case study 120
case studies 4
Caswell, G 56
causes of death 19
chaplaincy services 30

Cheyne–Stokes respiration 46
chronic disease trajectory 65–6
Church of England 34
CINAHL 147
clinical experience 151–2
clinical uncertainty 145–7
Cochrane Library 148
collaboration 93
comfort-focused approach 9
communication 4, 48–9
communication skills 32
compassionate engagement 30
complex patient needs
    delirium 88
    homelessness 89
    learning disabilities 90–1
    overview 87–8
complexity
    in care 83–7
    case study 82, 85–7
    overview 82–3
continuity 92–3
conversations about ACPs 111–14
coordination 16
courses 96–7
Covid-19 pandemic 19, 20–1
Critical Appraisal Skills Programme (CASP) 149–50
cultural competence 34
culture 33–7
curative care 9

death certificate 18–19
decolonisation 35–6
delirium 45, 82, 88
dementia 21
dignity 70–1
DNACPR (Do Not Attempt Resuscitation) 45, 48,
        51, 105–6
dwindling trajectory 66–7
dying alone 56–7
dying person 45–6

eLearning for health 96
Elsie case study 51–2
emotional intelligence 98
end of life 7, 9–10
End of Life Care for All 96
End of Life Think Tank 103
enduring power of attorney 107
equitable access 12

euthanasia 116
evidence-based practice 137–40
   clinical uncertainty 145–7
   jigsaw 150–2
expertise 151–2

Faith at End of Life (PHE) 34–5
family perspectives 52–4
fatigue 45, 78
Finucane, A 94–5
Flynn case study 95–6
focused questions 145–9
frailty 67
Future Nurse Standards 137–8, 144
FutureLearn 96

generalist palliative care 10–12
Gerber, K, 140–1
Gethin case study 120–1
good death 49–52
Grace case study 85–6
Grainger, K. 33
guidelines 138

Hawthorne, D 31
healthcare professionals 110–11
hellomynameis campaign 33
Hinduism 34
holistic biopsychosocial perspective 63
homelessness 89
hospice at home 12, 21
hospice care 12, 13
Hospice UK 47, 48
hospital deaths 56
Humanism 34
hydration changes 45
hyperactive delirium 88
hypoactive delirium 88

inequality 36–7
informal carers 122–4
integrated care 92
Ipsos Mori survey 42–3
Isaac case study 7
Islam 34

Jacob, Rita and Marc case study 67–8
James Lind Alliance 143

Kai case study 102, 114–16

lasting power of attorney (LPA) 107
learning disabilities 90–1
life-limiting illnesses
   case study 62, 67
   dignity 70–1
   disease trajectories 64–8
   fatigue 78
   functional changes 69–70
   health and 63–4
   overview 62–3
   pain assessment 76–8

   promotion of functioning 74
   quality of life 71
   rehabilitative model 72–4
   symptom management 74–5
'likely to be dying' 44
locations of care 55–6
Luis case study 28

Mannix, K 46, 103, 112
Marc case study 75
Mari case study 89
Marie Curie 90
media portrayals 42–3
Medical Certificate of Cause of Death (MCCD) 18–19
MEDLINE 147
Mental Capacity Act 2021 108
Mitchell, W 62
motor neurone disease (MND) 114–16
Mr and Mrs Fitzwilliam scenario 126
Mrs Zhang scenario 83, 84–5
multimorbidity 68
Murray, S 68

naive culturalism 34
National Institute for Health and Care Excellence
   (NICE) 138
nausea and vomiting 78
Nightingale, F 8, 138
Nitizimira, C 35
No Barriers Here 90
normality of dying 42–4
nurses' role 14–18
Nursing and Midwifery Council (NMC) 3–4, 25–6
Nursing Times 97
nursing verification of death 47–8
nutrition changes 45

O'Connor, M 56
Office for National Statistics (ONS) 19
ordinary power of attorney (OPA) 107

pain assessment 76–8
palliative care
   care settings 7
   explanation of 8–10
   generalist and specialist 10–12
   overview 1–2
participatory learning 96
Pask, S 87–8
patients
   ACPs 110
   preferences 152
person-centred care 24–6
   limitations of 26–7
person-centred goal-setting 72–3
person in the patient case study 27–8
personal appearance 29
personal care 45
personal development plans (PDPs) 4
personalised care 94
personhood 28–9
PICO framework 145–6

place of death 19–20, 20t
planning for palliative care
    conversations about 111–14
    overview 102–3
    planning ahead 103–4
Porter, l, 142
power of attorney 107–8, 115
preferred place of care 109
Price, B 26
proactive advice 129
professional relationships 129
progressive illnesses 28
psychological factors 84, 86

qualitative evidence synthesis 142
qualitative research 140–1
quality of life 71
quantitative research 141–2

Rachel case study 82
rallying 44, 46
randomised controlled trials (RCTs) 141–2
Recommended Summary Plan for Emergency Care
        and Treatment (ReSPECT) 106–7
Registered Nurse Verification of Expected Adult Death 47–8
relationship-centred care 27
research
    appraising 149–50
    evidence-based practice 137–40, 143–5
    overview 137
    questions 143
    types of 140–2
    using 144–5, 150–1
resilience 98
Resuscitation Council 106–7
revalidation 96
Richardson, H 72
Rietjens, J 110–11
rituals 34–5
Rodríguez-Pratt, A 71
Roman Catholicism 34
Rosa case study 62, 72–3

Saunders, C 7, 13–14, 15, 48, 78
scenarios 4
Seacole, M 8

searching 148
secretions 46
Sekse Review 15–18
self-care 95–6, 97–8
service provision issues 84, 86
signs of dying 44–6
skin changes 46
sleeping 45
social care 56
social factors 84, 86
specialist palliative care 10–12, 94–5
SPICE framework 146
spiritual assessment tools 30–1
spiritual distress 30
spiritual factors 84, 86
spirituality 29–31
St Christopher's Hospice 13–14
St Mary's Hospital 13
stakeholders 92t
Standards of Proficiency for Registered Nurses 3–4
Stephan case study 137, 144
student nurse responsibilities 114–16
Sue case study 52–4
support 17
symptom management 74–5
systematic reviews 142–3

terminal illness trajectory 64–5
therapeutic relationships 31–3
Tiberini, R 72
time constraints 17
top tips 58
total pain 15, 78
traditions 34–5
treatment escalation plans (TEPs) 103, 106
tri-morbidity 89

unexpected deaths 41–2

verification of death 47–8
Vickova, K 152

wellbeing, promotion of 62
what matters to you 103–4, 130–2
what's needed 16–17
World Health Organisation 8, 92–3